GAY AND LESBIAN YOUTH

THE SERIES IN CLINICAL AND COMMUNITY PSYCHOLOGY

CONSULTING EDITORS
Charles D. Spielberger and Irwin G. Sarason

Auerbach and Stolberg Crisis Intervention with Children and Families
Burchfield Stress: Psychological and Physiological Interactions
Burstein and Loucks Rorschach's Test: Scoring and Interpretation
Cohen and Ross Handbook of Clinical Psychobiology and Pathology, volume 1
Cohen and Ross Handbook of Clinical Psychobiology and Pathology, volume 2
Diamant Male and Female Homosexuality: Psychological Approaches
Froehlich, Smith, Draguns, and Hentschel Psychological Processes in Cognition and Personality
Hobfoll Stress, Social Support, and Women
Janisse Pupillometry: The Psychology of the Pupillary Response
Krohne and Laux Achievement, Stress, and Anxiety
London Personality: A New Look at Metatheories
London The Modes and Morals of Psychotherapy, Second Edition
Manschreck and Kleinman Renewal in Psychiatry: A Critical Rational Perspective
Morris Extraversion and Introversion: An Interactional Perspective
Muñoz Depression Prevention: Research Directions
Olweus Aggression in the Schools: Bullies and Whipping Boys
Reitan and Davison Clinical Neuropsychology: Current Status and Applications
Rickel, Gerrard, and Iscoe Social and Psychological Problems of Women: Prevention and Crisis Intervention
Rofé Repression and Fear: A New Approach to the Crisis in Psychotherapy
Savin-Williams Gay and Lesbian Youth: Expressions of Identity
Smoll and Smith Psychological Perspectives in Youth Sports
Spielberger and Diaz-Guerrero Cross-Cultural Anxiety, volume 1
Spielberger and Diaz-Guerrero Cross-Cultural Anxiety, volume 2
Spielberger and Diaz-Guerrero Cross-Cultural Anxiety, volume 3
Spielberger and Diaz-Guerrero Cross-Cultural Anxiety, volume 4
Spielberger and Sarason Stress and Anxiety, volume 1
Sarason and Spielberger Stress and Anxiety, volume 2
Sarason and Spielberger Stress and Anxiety, volume 3
Spielberger and Sarason Stress and Anxiety, volume 4
Spielberger and Sarason Stress and Anxiety, volume 5
Sarason and Spielberger Stress and Anxiety, volume 6
Sarason and Spielberger Stress and Anxiety, volume 7
Spielberger, Sarason, and Milgram Stress and Anxiety, volume 8
Spielberger, Sarason, and Defares Stress and Anxiety, volume 9
Spielberger and Sarason Stress and Anxiety, volume 10: A Sourcebook of Theory and Research
Spielberger, Sarason, and Defares Stress and Anxiety, volume 11
Spielberger, Sarason, and Strelau Stress and Anxiety, volume 12
Strelau, Farley, and Gale The Biological Bases of Personality and Behavior, volume 1: Theories, Measurement Techniques, and Development
Strelau, Farley, and Gale The Biological Bases of Personality and Behavior, volume 2: Psychophysiology, Performance, and Applications
Suedfeld Psychology and Torture
Ulmer On the Development of a Token Economy Mental Hospital Treatment Program
Williams and Westermeyer Refugee Mental Health in Resettlement Countries

IN PREPARATION

Diamant Homosexual Issues in the Workplace
Fischer The Science of Psychotherapy
Reisman A History of Clinical Psychology
Spielberger and Vagg The Assessment and Treatment of Test Anxiety
Spielberger, Sarason, Strelau, and Brebner Stress and Anxiety, volume 13
Spielberger, Sarason, Kulcsár and Van Heck Stress and Anxiety, volume 14

GAY AND LESBIAN YOUTH: EXPRESSIONS OF IDENTITY

Ritch C. Savin-Williams
Cornell University

⬤HEMISPHERE PUBLISHING CORPORATION
A member of the Taylor & Francis Group
New York   Washington   Philadelphia   London

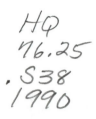

HQ
76.25
.S38
1990

GAY AND LESBIAN YOUTH: Expressions of Identity

1 2 3 4 5 6 7 8 9 0   B R B R   9 8 7 6 5 4 3 2 1 0

This book was set in Times Roman by Hemisphere Publishing Corporation. The editors were Amy Lyles Wilson, Deena Williams Newman, and Deborah Klenotic; the production supervisor was Peggy M. Rote; and the typesetter was Phoebe Carter. Cover design by Debra Eubanks Riffe. Printing and binding by Braum-Brumfield, Inc..

A CIP catalog record for this book is available from the British Library.

Library of Congress Cataloging-in-Publication Data

Savin-Williams, Ritch C.
   Gay and lesbian youth: expressions of identity / Ritch C. Savin-Williams
      p. cm. — (The Series in clinical and community psychology)
      Includes bibliographical references.
   1. Gay youth—Psychology.   I. Title   II. Series.
HQ76.25.S38   1990
306.76' 6' 0835—dc20   *89-26780*
                                                                CIP

ISBN 1-56032-037-0
ISSN 0146-0846

To Jim, for our life that we share.

Contents

Preface

This book addresses a recent theme in research and programs that focus on the life period of adolescence, "growing up forgotten." The writer cited most often on this topic, Joan Lipsitz (1977), identified the "forgotten" to be "normal," early adolescents. I depart from this concept in two ways. I include the whole period of adolescence, and restrict my scope to youths who are considered "abnormal" and "invisible" because of their sexual orientation.

Normal adolescence is no longer as forgotten, underresearched, or underserviced by social scientists or health care providers as it once was—aside from select populations such as youths of color or those below the poverty line (Savin-Williams, 1987a). For example, the Society for Research in Adolescence (SRA) has increased its membership from a dozen charter members in mid-1984 to more than 1,000 by the end of 1989. The field is blessed with half a dozen journals that have the terms *adolescence* or *youth* in their title. It is extremely rare, however, to discover SRA members who publish articles that are devoted to the study of gay and lesbian youth, the forgotten and invisible focus of this book.

During the last decade my scholarly efforts have been primarily directed toward issues of personality and social development during the adolescent years. The research reported in this book continued my interest in the psychological well-being of youth—in this case, lesbian and gay youth. Two outcome variables were explored: (a) feelings of self-worth and (b) the degree to which an individual acknowledges to the self and select others his or her sexual orientation. The recognition and expression of their most intimate secret is, perhaps more than any other single factor, intimately connected with psychological health during the adolescence of lesbian and gay individuals.

Several findings from a 6-year longitudinal study of self-esteem that I conducted among adolescents 12 to 18 years of age are particularly important for this book.[1] Most adolescents maintained a relatively stable level of self-esteem during this reputedly traumatic time in the life course. Most appeared to possess a baseline or core level of self-esteem from which temporal or contextual fluctuations, usually relatively mild, formed. Some youths had extremely stable

---

[1]See published reports by Savin-Williams and Demo (1983a, 1983b, 1984), Savin-Williams and Jaquish (1981), and Demo (1985).

levels of self-feelings regardless of where they were, who they were with, or what they were doing. A few others, on the other hand, were wildly oscillating—perhaps the adolescents usually encountered by clinicians and members of the media. For this relatively small number of youths, self-feelings at one moment were relatively independent of those at the next moment.

In the midst of considering my next research pursuit, I discovered theoretical speculations that puzzled and then infuriated me. Foremost among these was the perspective that gay males and lesbians, by definition, must have deficient levels of self-esteem. The cause was projected to be either developmental handicaps that resulted in both homosexuality and self-loathing or an internalization of the anti-gay values and attitudes of the external, homophobic world. Here was a topic that contained the unique combination of qualities rarely acknowledged in my profession—the scholarly interest and personal investment that sustain research endeavors after one has achieved the luxury and security of tenure in a university system.

This book is a presentation of my initial research in this field. First, theoretical positions on self-esteem and coming out among gay men and lesbians, and the empirical evidence for these assumptions, are reviewed. These are followed by discussion of my study on self-esteem and coming out in a sample of gay and lesbian youths. The study is unique because of the adolescent population studied and the attention it gave to variations within the gay and lesbian sample.

The research would never have been possible without the help of five research assistants. Their knowledge, critical insights, and friendship networks proved invaluable. Andrea Butt, from upstate New York, and Rala Massey, from rural Mississippi, were the first to volunteer their efforts. They critiqued the initial research instrument and formulated new independent variables. Later, Beth Burlingame, a psychology major, Jay Coburn, a gay activist, and Richard Goldberg, an artist and dancer, joined us.

My appreciation is also extended to the individuals and organizations (noted in Chapter 4) who assisted in the research effort; to the reviewers who commented on earlier drafts; to Vicki Griffin, who typed the many permutations of the manuscript; and, of course, to the 317 individuals who gave of their time to provide the data for this study.

Ritch C. Savin-Williams

GAY AND LESBIAN YOUTH

1

Forgotten and Invisible

OVERVIEW

A forgotten, invisible minority in North America today is the gay or lesbian adolescent. This condition promises to change as an increasing number of adolescents are exploring and expressing sexual behaviors and identities beyond the heterosexual ones that are traditionally assumed and bestowed by society. It is my hope that the legacy of this volume will be the reduction of this invisibility to social scientists and health care providers, to gay and lesbian communities, and to gay and lesbian youths themselves.

Homosexuality is both a personal and social issue with potent developmental significance:

> *The cumulative effects of being either an invisible or outcast segment of society are often that sexual minority youth feel bad about themselves, have a poor self-image and low self-esteem, and more than other teenagers, feel totally alone. (Vergara, 1983/1984, p. 23)*

The negative stereotypes of homosexuality prevalent in our society are reinforced by cultural forces such as the media, law, religion, and tradition, and those in a youth's immediate social world, that is, family members and adolescent peers. Images of what others believe it means to be gay are frequently voiced and perpetuated through "fag" and "dyke" jokes and demands to be gender appropriate in all aspects of life. Through an almost automatic association, homosexuality has become a stigma for even well-intentioned, reasonable youth and adults. As a result, for gay and lesbian youth this "stigma threatens both self-esteem and one's sense of identity by denying the social and emotional validation upon which those constructs are built" (Hammersmith, 1987, p. 176). Most youths are raised in heterosexual families, associate in heterosexual peer groups, and are educated in heterosexual institutions. Youth who are not heterosexual often feel they have little option except to pass as "heterosexually normal." The fact that they must hide their sexual orientation makes it assume a global significance to them considerably beyond necessary proportions.

Yet, to many, lesbian and gay youth do not exist. If families discover or are told of "peculiar behaviors or inclinations," the accused adolescents may be viewed as homosexually behaving youths temporarily detained from their destination as heterosexual adults. Gay and lesbian adolescents are faced with both a hostile and an unbelieving world. They are told, "You can't be a homosexual and I won't allow it." For those who discover the truthfulness and inevitability of their homosexuality and decide to contradict their previously assumed sexual identity, there are few sources of psychological, social, or legal assistance.

At a recent conference on gay and lesbian youth, many of the speakers noted that the paucity of research on gay and lesbian adolescents is appalling. Yet, few of

1

those present, including those who spoke out most forcefully, had in fact conducted empirical research with gay or lesbian youth.[1] In general, social scientists and health care providers have been hesitant to confront the stigmatic, legal, and moral issues involved with studying or assisting lesbian and gay minors (Robertson, 1981). Perhaps they fear the label of "guilty by association" and experience the unique dread of stereotypes that are usually applied to those who are involved with youth (e.g., pedophile). Theo Sandfort noted during a recent speaking tour of the United States that these negative reactions are usually more severe in this country than in other, more sex-positive societies such as the Netherlands. Even those who are most concerned with issues of homosexuality appear to assume that this sexual orientation is a prerogative only of adulthood.

Gay and lesbian organizations have also been reticent to assist the young gay or lesbian adolescent, perhaps because they fear the issue is too controversial (a disguised attempt to "recruit" young people) and complex (the social, legal, and economic status of dependent, minor youth) or because they lack the personnel, knowledge, and funds to offer support (D'Emilio, 1983; Robinson, 1984). Robinson (1984) noted,

> Whether due to inadequate professional knowledge, fear of jeopardizing professional positions, or simple lack of interest, personnel in youth-serving agencies and school districts (many of whom are gay themselves) have, for the most part, not been willing to speak out on behalf of gay youth. (p. 14)

But gay and lesbian youth are also frequently invisible to themselves. This is due, in part, to problems for oppressed minorities inherent in American society that values so highly uniformity and conformity. Thus, it is difficult to recognize and affirm "deviancy" in oneself. This failure to come forth compounds the difficulty of finding lesbian and gay youth as research participants, thus amplifying their invisibility. As a result, social scientists either ignore them in their research or rely on retrospective data-gathering techniques that ask gay and lesbian adults to reflect on their adolescence to recall important events, feelings, and relationships. Yet, recall-data methodologies make particular and often debatable assumptions concerning the accuracy of adult memories of childhood sexual feelings and behaviors (Boxer & Cohler, 1989; Ross, 1980).

SEXUAL ORIENTATION, SEXUAL BEHAVIOR, AND SEXUAL IDENTITY

Self-Label

An initial difficulty is defining who and what a homosexual is, both to the adolescent and to others, especially the family. This is not an easy task during this age because in general although adolescents are more likely to experience cross-orientation sexual contact than are adults, they are less likely to define themselves as homosexual individuals. Only 1 of 1,067 youths in a recent representative sample of adolescents (Coles & Stokes, 1985) checked the "homosexual" identity

---

[1]A notable exception is Remafedi's (1987a, 1987b) recent publications.

box. Yet, 5% reported that they had engaged in homosexual behavior during adolescence. In a 1985 survey of 356 high school students ages 16 to 18 enrolled in
Cornell University's Summer College, only 3 labeled themselves as bisexual/
homosexual; 5 rated themselves as "more than incidentally homosexual" and 15
as "incidentally homosexual" on the Kinsey Heterosexual-Homosexual Rating
Scale (Savin-Williams, 1989c). The next year, of 176 youths surveyed during the
same program only 1 student expressed same-sex sexual attraction; another 4
replied "both sexes equally." Behaviorally, 12 reported past and 8 reported current
"casual" homosexual encounters; 3 reported genital–genital homosexual contact
in their past. Thus, youth are far more likely to "admit" to homosexual acts than
to a homosexual identity.

It is unclear from the empirical research the degree to which cohort and/or
developmental effects determine an individual's labeling himself or herself as gay
or lesbian. Boxer and Cohler (1989) made the strong argument that because of past
research efforts, which were primarily cross-sectional studies of the remembered
past of gay and lesbian adults, little is known concerning either developmental
processes or cultural/historical effects on lesbian and gay adolescents. The argument here is for a developmental paradigm, without intending to negate or ignore
cohort effects. Indeed, it is probably easier to come out as a homosexual youth
today than it was for previous generations, who came into their adolescence before
the benchmark 1969 Stonewall encounter with the New York City police. If it were
possible to control or account for historical time, I believe developmental
differences in coming out would still emerge. With advancing age, especially after
the increase in sexual libido and cognitive abilities during pubescence, the equation
of sexual behavior and sexual identity becomes both easier and more
necessary.

Definitions

These issues reinforce the need to distinguish among the concepts sexual
orientation, sexual behavior, and sexual identity. A homosexual *sexual orientation*
consists of a preponderance of sexual or erotic feelings, thoughts, fantasies, and/or
behaviors desired with members of the same sex. It is present from an early age—
perhaps at conception (see Savin-Williams, 1987b). Homosexual activity or the
"homosexually stimulating experience" (Rigg, 1982) connotes *sexual behavior*
between members of the same sex. *Sexual identity,* by contrast, represents a
consistent, enduring self-recognition of the meanings that sexual orientation and
sexual behavior have for oneself. Although a public declaration of this status is not
inherently necessary for sexual identity, there must be some level of personal
recognition of this status. Affirmation, to varying degrees, may or may not
follow.

These definitions serve to illustrate the essential differences among sexual orientation, sexual behavior, and inner identity. Although it is likely that the three will
be somewhat or highly correlated, this may be more of a future adult than a
present adolescent reality. This issue is particularly crucial in reference to teenage
populations because it appears that many forms of sexual activity with partners
varying in age, sex, and other person variables are commonplace, regardless of
self-labeled or self-professed sexual orientation and identity.

The confusion is illustrated by two seemingly opposite facts: Some gay and lesbian adolescents are homosexual virgins and some heterosexual adolescents engage in extensive and prolonged homosexual behavior. Studies (Boxer, 1988; Remafedi, 1987a; Roesler & Deisher, 1972; G. Sanders, 1980) of gay and lesbian youths support the claim that some accept the self-label of gay/lesbian before they have had homosexual experiences. Among 118 youths who came to Chicago's Horizons Center, 9% of the boys and 6% of the girls had never experienced same-sex activity (Boxer, 1988). Manosevitz (1970) reported that 22% of his male sample were homosexual virgins during the ages of 13 to 17 years and 4% during the ages 18 to 24 years. In Hedblom's (1973) study, 66% of the female sample were homosexual virgins before age 15 years and 21% at age 20 years. Dank (1971) concluded,

> It is theoretically possible for someone to view himself as being homosexual but not engage in homosexual relations just as it is possible for someone to view himself as heterosexual but not engage in heterosexual relations. (p. 117)

On the other hand, clearly not all adolescents who engage in homosexual behavior would identify themselves as gay or lesbian. Kinsey, Pomeroy, and Martin (1948) found that

> between adolescence and 15 years of age about 1 male in 4 (27%) has some homosexual experience. The figures rise to 1 male in 3 in the later teens and appear to drop a bit in the early twenties. (p. 629)

Yet,

> 4 percent of the white males are exclusively homosexual throughout their lives, after the onset of adolescence. [Kinsey et al.'s emphasis] (p. 651)

In the Sorensen Report (1973), 5% of the boys and 6% of the girls ages 13 to 15 years responded positively to the statement "Have you had activity with another boy [girl] or with a grown man [woman] that resulted in sexual stimulation or satisfaction for either or both of you?" Among 16- to 19-year-olds the percentage of boys marking "yes" more than tripled to 17% while the proportion of girls remained at 6%. Saghir and Robins (1973) reported 23% of their heterosexual males had had homosexual contacts by age 15 years; Ramsey (1943), 31% by age 17 years; and Manosevitz (1970), 23% by age 17 years. Recent data (Fay, Turner, Klassen, & Gagnon, 1989) estimated the percentage somewhat lower: 20.3% of a national representative sample had had homosexual contact at some point during their lifetime.

Among females the percentages are smaller but in the same direction. In Kinsey, Pomeroy, Martin, and Gebhard's study (1953), by age 15 years 5% of the females had experienced homosexual contact and 2% were exclusively homosexual by sexual orientation. Ten percent of 160 women in a university dormitory had had homosexual encounters (Goode & Haber, 1977). Others (Manosevitz, 1970; Ramsey, 1943; Saghir & Robins, 1973; Sorensen, 1973) have reported similar statistics and conclusions.

Malyon (1981) speculated that about 9 in 10 reports by youth of same-sex erotic interest are made by those predominantly heterosexual in orientation. However, Ross-Reynolds (1982, p. 70) concluded, "The majority of adolescents who engage in homosexual behavior do not continue this practice into adulthood. Conversely, as many as 31% of gay adults engaged in no homosexual behavior until they were out of high school." This quote illustrates the difficulty of equating homosexual behavior with either sexual orientation or identity.

Still, there is ample evidence that "pre-gay and pre-lesbian" adolescents are more likely than others to engage in homosexual behavior and to do so for a longer period of time. For example, Bell, Weinberg, and Hammersmith (1981a, 1981b) reported that 95% and 70% of their homosexual men and women, respectively, but only 20% and 6% of their heterosexual men and women, respectively, had been sexually aroused by a member of the same sex before they reached 19 years of age. Only 2% and zero, respectively, of heterosexual men and women rated their preadult sexual behaviors as predominantly homosexual, as opposed to 56% and 44% of the homosexual men and women, respectively, who so reported. In another sample of gay men and women (Saghir & Robins, 1969; Saghir, Robins, & Walbran, 1969), 87% had had homosexual contacts before the age of 19 years. In a West German sample of women, 52% had had homosexual contacts by the same age (Schafer, 1977). Compared with heterosexuals, Manosevitz (1970) noted, the homosexuals in his sample had been more sexually active prior to adolescence. "They seemed to start earlier, and the direction of their activities was towards same-sexed partners. . . . Then many shifted to male and female partners during adolescence and early adulthood" (p. 401). During childhood (5 to 9 years) 41% of the homosexual males had had same-sex sexual activity, and this proportion steadily increased to 59% during preadolescence (10 to 12 years), 70% during adolescence (13 to 17 years), and 96% during late adolescence and youth (18 to 24 years). The percentages of heterosexuals who had engaged in homosexual behavior were considerably lower and decreased rather than increased after preadolescence: 5% during childhood, 25% during preadolescence, 15% during adolescence, and 5% during late adolescence (Manosevitz, 1970). In a study of gay males between the ages of 16 and 22 years, Roesler and Deisher (1972) reported that the majority described early, prepubertal homosexual activity (e.g., mutual body exploration or curiosity-based sex play). Of 29 homosexual or bisexual males, ages 15 to 19 years, 28 had had past homosexual encounters, but most of these had occurred during early adolescence (Remafedi, 1987a). Van Wyk and Geist (1984) documented among Kinsey's (1948) sample that the more elevated the homosexual score, the greater the likelihood of prepubertal sexual contact with boys or men for homosexual men.

Thus there can be little doubt that not only does homosexual behavior occur during adolescence, it may also be quite prevalent. Such behavior, however, may or may not be indicative of a homosexual orientation or identification. Given the complexity of whether one defines homosexuality by reference to orientation, behavior, or self-awareness and the fact that many teens experience a diversity of sexual behaviors and an emerging sexual identity over a period of several years, a process that may not be completed until young adulthood, it is difficult to assess the prevalence of a homosexual orientation among adolescents. Despite this handicap, it is abundantly clear that gay and lesbian youth exist during childhood and adolescence—with or without homosexual behavior and/or a homosexual identity. Understanding of these issues is enhanced with a cross-cultural perspective.

Cross-Cultural Research

Anthropological research documents that homosexual behavior exists in most cultures when sufficient detail of sexual behavior is recorded. Ford and Beach's (1951, p. 143) early review is frequently cited as sufficient evidence for the universality of homosexual behavior: "The cross-cultural and cross-species comparisons presented in this chapter combine to suggest that a biological tendency for inversion of sexual behavior is inherent in most if not all mammals including the human species." In various human cultures adolescent homosexual behavior may be viewed as necessary (because the sexes are separated), as preparatory for heterosexual activity (to learn about sex), as giving ritualized status such as manhood (a semen implant for masculinity to thrive), as playful acting out of the increased sexual libido derived from pubertal hormones, or (rarely) as an expression of a life-long sexual orientation.

The evidence for universal homosexuality as a sexual orientation is less secure. Whitam (1983; Whitam & Mathy, 1987) concluded from his study of homosexuality in the United States, Guatemala, Brazil, and the Philippines and his review of the anthropological evidence that homosexuality is prevalent to about the same degree in all societies and has remained stable over time. In addition, homosexual persons in different societies tend to resemble each other with respect to certain behavioral interests and occupational choices. Social norms do not apparently impede or facilitate the emergence of homosexuality:

> Homosexuality is not created by social structural arrangements but is rather a fundamental form of human sexuality acted out in different cultural settings. . . . It does seem clear from the cross-cultural perspective that societies do not create homosexuals. Their emergence appears to be beyond the power of any society to control. (Whitam, 1983, pp. 207 and 209)

Although homosexuality is considered by some to be universal cross-culturally, it is clearly not documented in all cultures. This is perhaps due to the secretive nature in which it is carried out and the difficulty of satisfactorily applying a common definition to or empirically assessing the abstract construct of homosexuality as a sexual orientation. One extreme view is that of Gadpaille (1980), who concluded that homosexuality as a preferred sexual expression after adolescence is universally deemed deviant, although he noted that in some cultures homosexuality has been given an institutional role and its stigmatization has been moderated.

Because homosexual behavior is more clearly demarcated and observable, it is more frequently documented cross-culturally. Clearly, societies vary in how they react to the emergence of homosexual behavior among their adolescent citizens, including the degree to which they allow it to be overtly manifested and stigmatized. Some cultures celebrate homosexual behavior among their adolescents, perhaps even proscribing it (e.g., Sambia in New Guinea [Herdt, 1981]). Two-thirds of modern tribes in South America consider adolescent homosexuality to be both normal and acceptable (noted in Tannahill, 1980). Other cultures tolerate/ignore homosexual behavior or, if it is brought into public view, actively discourage it.

A classic example of the latter is the English public school system. In the late 19th century it kept upper class boys secluded from girls in a monastic fashion through most of childhood and adolescence (Tannahill, 1980). After the occurrence of the Oscar Wilde "scandal," many well-bred Englishmen came to recognize that Eton, Harrow, and Winchester were "breeding grounds" for homosexual behavior and that some adolescent boys continued the behavior into adulthood. Lax laws against sodomy were then enforced with moral conviction.

Southern Italian culture tends to allow homosexual experimentation among adolescent males (Dall'orto, 1987). Because of its Catholic heritage, there is an obsession within Italian culture to prevent premarital and extramarital heterosexual activities, yet because "boys married somewhat late and their poverty precluded access to prostitutes, a homosexual outlet has always been regarded as a good alternative for teen-agers to have fun—especially when the homosexual partner handed over a small bribe for the 'service'" (p. 28).

All adults are assumed to be heterosexual in Italian culture; deviations from this norm are tolerated through religious and legal silence. But with the modern increasing visibility of homosexuality and homosexual behavior, cultural shifts are evident. For example, in a recent *New York Times* "About Men" article, Youman noted that Italian men no longer publicly walk hand in hand or arm in arm. He questioned, "Has the emergence of homosexual men from their closets had, as a by-product, a chilling effect on heterosexual males' willingness to be seen touching one another in public?" (Youman, 1985, p. 74). This was, he felt, a tragic loss, one that he experienced directly when his 17-year-old son stiffened when he touched him.

These studies are promising in their attempts to describe the incidence and prevalence of both homosexual activity and homosexual identity during adolescence, as well as the relationship between the two. Investigators across cultures seldom agree on identifiable, specific variables that accurately predict a young person's ultimate sexual behavior or orientation, although the existence of many have been a source of speculation with varying degrees of supporting research evidence. For example, inferences concerning an adolescent's sexuality are frequently based on certain "suspicious" gender-atypical behaviors, dress, and mannerisms. Of deep concern to some has been explaining the prevalence of homosexual behavior during adolescence.

Explanations for Adolescent Homosexual Behavior

Great effort, primarily anecdotal in nature, has been made to account for the relatively high frequency of homosexual experiences among teenagers. Some (Glasser, 1977; Rigg, 1982) have argued that sexual experimentation with same-sex peers occurs because exploration of bodies and reactions is more familiar and therefore less threatening than similar heterosexual physical contact. Others (e.g., Sorensen, 1973) have postulated that reassurance is gained from mutual comparisons of size, shape, and sensations associated with changing bodies and sex organs; still others (e.g., Chng, 1980) have viewed these "transient homosexual activities" as the product of typical adolescent crushes, hero worship, and intimate same-sex friendships. Glasser (1977) proposed that few of the adolescents who have homoerotic impulses or behaviors ever become homosexual. Rather, he argued that normal boys engage in homosexual behavior to release sexual drives thwarted by parents who are "protecting" their adolescent daughters.

Similarly, Robinson (1980) viewed the psychodynamics of adolescent sexuality as frequently including homosexual behavior which, under normal circumstances, is gradually replaced by heterosexual development. A "normal" homosexual stage in early adolescence was thought to be comparable to sleep disturbances or enure-sis: Teenagers were expected to have these developmental problems and then out-grow them. This view was willing to entertain the possibility that homosexual experiences may even be necessary for some heterosexual youths. Typically, this so-called normal homosexual stage was presumed to last until early or middle adolescence, followed by a move to heterosexuality. One fear was that if homosex-ual attachments became intense and exclusive then more overt homosexual activity was considered likely with a concomitant absence of motivation to advance to heterosexual activity. Thus, it was assumed that a homosexual sexual orientation was an achieved status, obtained through social conditioning or circumstances. Throughout these writings, it was emphasized that adolescents *must* make the choice to progress to heterosexuality.

Adolescent homosexual activities have thus been frequently viewed as a "nor-mal phase" of adult heterosexual development that "need cause no anxiety that they are the harbingers of lifelong homosexuality" (Rigg, 1982, p. 828). This form of denial may be soothing to concerned and frightened parents, but it may potentially be a source of self-denial if not great anxiety to the teenager who is becoming aware of a developing homosexual identity that does not fit these expec-tations. For such individuals, homosexuality is not experienced as a temporary phase but as a true identity.

Thus, it is crucial that social scientists, health care providers, parents, and youth are aware of the following empirical evidence:

1. Not all homosexual adolescents are sexually active,
2. Many homosexual adolescents are heterosexually active,
3. Many heterosexual adolescents are homosexually active,
4. The synchrony between sexual identity and sexual behavior is highly vari-able among adolescents,
5. Many of these issues evoke great stress and anxiety for adolescents of all sexual orientations.

Knowing whether a youth identifies himself or herself as gay or straight may not be helpful in assessing the incidence or frequency of homosexual behavior. Although an adolescent who self-identifies as homosexual is more likely than one who self-labels as heterosexual to have engaged in homosexual behavior (and at a higher frequency rate), such individuals may also be homosexual virgins and some self-labeled heterosexual youths may be quite homosexually active.

Perhaps less so than at any other age, an adolescent's stated sexual orientation may be of limited significance to the researcher, the health care provider, or the parent. Consequently, when developing research projects or educational health programs in which homosexual behavior is a critical consideration, it becomes particularly salient to consider all adolescents, not just those currently aware of a bisexual or homosexual identity.

PRIOR RESEARCH WITH LESBIAN AND GAY YOUTHS

Throughout this book it will be noted that there are relatively few published reports of lesbians and gay males that include adolescents and youths in the analysis. As a result, it is extremely difficult to know whether and how lesbian and gay youths differ from adult lesbians and gay males and among themselves (e.g., early vs. late adolescents). Most age comparisons have focused on contrasting the "aged homosexual" with other gay and lesbian adults (see books and articles by Berger, 1982; Friend, 1980; Gray & Dressel, 1985; Raphael & Robinson, 1980; Weinberg & Williams, 1974). Developmental studies are rare. Green's (1987) study is a notable exception with a select subpopulation of (effeminate) males. Reasons for their scarcity are easy to understand, given the desire for secrecy of most research participants. Longitudinal studies are extremely difficult to implement when the issue is so stigmatized that the subjects participate only with the promise of non-identification, which eliminates any opportunity for follow-up studies. As a result, previously reported studies of youths have been severely limited in scope (e.g., the age range of subjects is so narrow as to be of questionable value).

Perhaps the earliest study of gay youth is Roesler and Deisher's (1972) research with youths a full cohort older than the present research participants. It was conducted not for basic research purposes but to assist physicians and counselors who might want to intervene in the lives of prehomosexual boys. Of the 60 young males interviewed for 1 hour in Seattle, 40 were "introduced to us through acquaintances who knew the young men had homosexual experiences" (Roesler & Deisher, 1972, p. 1018). The rest were located in gay bars, beaches, parks, and the Selective Service (those dismissed or rejected from service). Little information is provided describing these youths aside from their sexual behavior, coming-out status, and socialization/counseling patterns. The age range was 16 to 22 years (M = 20 years); 62% considered themselves homosexual, 31% bisexual, and 7% undecided/heterosexual. Many had come out (73%), experienced a large number of homosexual encounters (median = 50), visited a psychiatrist (48%), and attempted suicide (31%).

Remafedi's (1987a, 1987b) 29 young men from Minneapolis and St. Paul ranged from 15 to 19 years of age (M = 18.3 years)[2] and were either homosexual (79%) or bisexual (21%). These subjects were recruited for the research project through newspaper and radio advertisements, a health department clinic, and referrals by participants. They were paid a small fee. Most were White (90%), middle class, and urban (80%). Two-thirds did not live with their parents and were employed. All were out to friends or family members, 72% had consulted a psychologist or psychiatrist, 58% were substance abusers, 34% had attempted suicide, and 31% had been hospitalized for mental health reasons. The mean age indicates that relatively few 15- or 16-year-olds were interviewed. The youths were divided into two groups, those under 18 years of age (n = 18) and those age 18 or 19 (n = 11). The younger group was significantly more likely to report psychosocial problems such as substance abuse, conflict with the law, hospitalization in a psychiatric unit, and dropping out of high school.

The Chicago Youth Project, conducted by Herdt, Boxer, and Irvin, is a just-completed study of coming out as a cultural rite of passage. Two hundred self-

---

[2]There appears to be a problem with either the mean age given or the stated makeup of the two groups. Remafedi divided his youths into two groups. If all 11 youths in the older group were the oldest possible (19 years old) and the younger group was the oldest composition possible (one 15-year-old and 17 17-year-olds) the mean for the sample would be 17.69 years. This is the oldest that the sample could be, given the author's (Remafedi, 1987b) published statement. Yet, the reported mean age is 18.3 years.

identified lesbian and gay adolescents, ages 14 to 21 years, from the Horizons youth group were interviewed. Boxer (1988) has focused on issues most germane to the current study: awareness of first same-sex attractions, fantasies, and sexual activity and the self-disclosure process. Irvin (1988), using several additional measures—the Klein Sexual Orientation Scale, the Symptom Checklist–90 index of symptomatology, and a self-esteem sentence completion test—is developing a typology of coping with same-sex attractions, behavior, fantasies, and social-emotional preferences among the Horizon youths.

The first two studies are clearly restricted in scope and were of limited usefulness for purposes of the present research. Data from the Chicago Youth Project will eventually be of greater significance for the variables reported in this book. Unfortunately, however, their data analyses, aside from preliminary reports based on a subset of the population, are in the initial stages. Because of the relatively few investigations of lesbian and gay youth, by necessity one must turn to evidence provided by retrospective accounts of adults as they reflect on their adolescence for empirical evidence of variables that are associated with or predict self-esteem and coming out. In regard to self-esteem, this strategy may not necessarily produce erroneous relationships if one accepts the view that self-esteem is essentially a stable characteristic of one's personality and thus not generally subject to high degrees of modification as the direct result of situational or environmental factors (Savin-Williams & Demo, 1984). Coming out, on the other hand, is a process that is by definition reactive to developmental as well as social and historical pressures. As such, retrospective accounts of coming out may be influenced by present life circumstances, memories, attitudes, and beliefs. Thus, the available literature must be viewed with caution in terms of its relevance for present populations of lesbian and gay youth.

An important limitation was placed on the literature reviewed in this book: Only research in which the participants were gay men, lesbians, or bisexuals is considered. This decision had no real impact in regard to coming out because there is clearly no comparable literature for straight youth—there is no need to "come out" as straight. There is, however, a large body of empirical studies that attempt to predict self-acceptance or self-esteem level based on almost any conceivable variable. This literature is not summarized in this book for several reasons. First, I did not want to assume that self-esteem is related to the tested variables in the same manner that has been empirically demonstrated with heterosexual populations. Perhaps the developmental trajectory of evolving a sense of self-worth among lesbian and gay youth is in some way unique. Second, I wanted to avoid the danger of posing straight youth as a control or comparison group. To do so would imply that gay and lesbian youth are normal or psychologically healthy only when they are similar to heterosexual youth. When they are not similar to heterosexual youth, then something must be wrong. Third, I was not willing to assume that I had sampled a "normal" or random subset of gay and lesbian youth. Therefore, it would be difficult to operationally define a comparable heterosexual sample. Thus, for both professional and political reasons, assumptions and implications of straight versus gay research were avoided.

In the next two chapters basic issues regarding self-esteem (Chapter 2) and coming out (Chapter 3) are reviewed. The invisibility and neglect of gay and lesbian youth suggested in this chapter are reexamined in Chapter 10.

2

The Alleged Self-Hatred of Gays

OVERVIEW

Psychologists' and sociologists' interest in issues of youth development escalated during the neo-Darwinian period in the early 1900s when evolutionary concepts were applied not only to the genesis of species but also to the ontogeny of human development. The biological changes that define adolescence were perceived as significant because they represent to the individual and the species that supreme moment in time when the individual becomes capable of, and perhaps also willing to, reproduce and disperse his or her genes to the world.[1] Thus, youth were G. Stanley Hall's (1904) hope for the future of the human species and Friedrich Nietzsche's (1961) hope for the evolution of the historical Superman.

The physical and sexual changes that define pubescence are associated with increased cognitive skills and abilities. These allow a youth to construct a self beyond the simple bounds of the past to include what one is as well as what one might become. These new reflective cognitive skills, in combination with the sexual and physical pubertal changes, result in an increased concern with the self as is, a conception of what the self should be, the all too apparent discrepancy between the two, and a need to validate the self to significant others.

A number of theorists built on these themes of self development during adolescence, for example, William James (1890) and Erik Erikson (1959) in psychology and George Herbert Mead (1934), Morris Rosenberg (1965, 1979), and Stanley Coopersmith (1967) in sociology. Sociologists expanded the psychologists' attention beyond the physical changes of puberty and cognition to a concern with the importance of the social contexts that influence patterns of self-conception. As the individual moves out of the family and into the larger, peer-dominated external world, he or she confronts societal expectations of what is appropriate or inappropriate behavior (Savin-Williams & Berndt, 1990). The self, once protected and secured during the childhood years, may feel more vulnerable and in a greater state of flux than at any other time in the life course. Regardless of theoretical or disciplinary orientation, the self is frequently portrayed as subject to alterations and doubts during adolescence.

Self-concept is not a simple notion, and social scientists have certainly not ignored its presence among either heterosexual or homosexual populations. One aspect of the self-concept that is of vital importance to youth is the self-evaluation dimension, frequently referred to as self-esteem. Perhaps no other aspect of human existence, with the exception of intelligence and social class, has received such

---

[1]These themes are developed in considerably more detail in *Adolescence: An Ethological Perspective* (Savin-Williams, 1987a) and a chapter in *The Biology of Adolescent Behavior and Development* (Savin-Williams & Weisfeld, 1989).

extensive coverage from both psychologists and sociologists. This may reflect our American high acclaim for individual competencies, such as being happy (self-esteem), smart (IQ), and rich (social class). In particular, during the years of adolescence developmental psychologists and sociologists have focused on feelings of self-worth, perhaps because IQ and social class appear to be beyond the ability of psychologists to control ("smart" is subject to one's genetic heritage and "rich" to one's familial heritage). This concern by professionals with the developmental importance of self-esteem is frequently shared by youth.

In mainstream developmental psychology, a central issue in self-evaluation research is what correlates with or predicts self-esteem during the adolescent and young adult years. Typically, self-esteem refers to the global evaluation that an individual makes and customarily maintains with regard to the self, independent of context (Rosenberg, 1979). This approval or disapproval toward the self is the experienced dimension of self-esteem that can best be assessed by self-report measures (Savin-Williams & Jaquish, 1981).

When applied to lesbian and gay youth, however, this research concern has been preempted by a greater focus on tracing the etiological connection between self-evaluation and sexual orientation. For example, it is not uncommon for psychoanalytic theorists to attribute to homosexuality a wide range of neurotic problems that relate to how individuals evaluate their self-image. Because of their sexual orientation, it is believed that homosexual persons have a developmental history of serious personality disturbances that result in self-doubts, sadistic and masochistic behavior, and suicidal gestures (Romm, 1965). This connection is due to very early experiences with the parents who become objects of erotic stimulation and hence sources of identification. These dually contribute to self-hatred and sexual inversion (Bell, 1975).

From a sociological theoretical perspective, Hoffman (1968) noted that for the homosexual male self-esteem depends on two factors: his internalized values and the reflected appraisals he receives from others, especially his parents. Self-esteem is low because he participates in behavior—intimate relations with other males—deemed deviant by the general culture. Spada (1979) reported that gay men who are unhappy generally attributed their condition not to their homosexuality per se but to the way society treats gay people. This view proposes that self-evaluation through childhood, adolescence, and adulthood is dependent in large measure on an acceptance of the values and attitudes of the social world.

These two theoretical perspectives have been the major conceptual explanations for the low sense of self-worth purported to be characteristic of lesbian and gay youth. They have fostered the stereotype of the homosexual as an unhappy individual living a lonely, depressed life. Supposedly the gay man despises his sexual partners as much as he despises himself and the lesbian constantly craves praise and affection from others, reflecting the reality of her inferior life-style (Davis, 1985; Dorian, 1965). Those who possess low self-esteem fear intimacy and experience loneliness; they turn to homosexuality to find partial relief (Thompson, 1973). Furthermore, we are asked to believe that it is inevitable that the homosexual individual will devaluate the self either because of long-standing developmental handicaps or because of a homophobic social world. The homosexual youth must, by definition, hate himself or herself. These stereotyped, traditional views are held by too many lay and professional, heterosexual and homosexual individuals.

Each of the two theories is briefly explored in this chapter. Then, research comparing homosexual and heterosexual self-esteem is examined to empirically test the theoretical conclusion of both psychoanalysis and sociological theory: Homosexual individuals have low self-esteem. If this conclusion is accurate, then further elaborations of the two theories should be pursued; if it is not accurate, then the theories should be repaired or one can conclude that the research question as framed and tested is not particularly useful and perhaps counterproductive.

PSYCHOANALYTIC PERSPECTIVES

Psychoanalytic theorists generally integrate sexuality and other aspects of personality; deviance in one arena increases the likelihood of deviance in the other. In *Homosexuality: Disease or Way of Life?*, Bergler (1956) answered the question he posed, "Is sex or the whole personality sick in homosexuals?", with a resounding "BOTH." He then proceeded to list the ways. For some psychoanalysts all problems of self-affect, for example, emotional isolation and intolerable loneliness, are inherent in the contradictions and defects of the homosexual condition (Bieber, 1965). This view neglects, and certainly distorts, Sigmund Freud's position that all individuals are born constitutionally with a bisexual potentiality and his generally compassionate understanding of homosexuality. The latter is reflected in a letter he wrote to a distraught mother of a gay son: "Homosexuality is assuredly no advantage but it is nothing to be ashamed of, no vice, no degradation, it cannot be classified as an illness; we consider it to be a variation of the sexual function produced by a certain arrest of sexual development" (Freud, 1935, p. 786). He felt that it was both cruel and unjust to consider homosexuality a crime.

Although there are many varieties of psychoanalytic theory, Kwawer (1980) noted that psychoanalysis is frequently portrayed as a cohesive orthodoxy that has neither diversity nor the capacity to change. Freud himself proposed several major theories concerning the origins of homosexuality that are at the same time both contradictory and complementary (Lewes, 1988). However, two primary etiological defects leading to homosexuality appear repeatedly in the psychoanalytic literature: developmental anomalies occurring during either the preoedipal or oedipal period (Ovesey & Woods, 1980). The first became popular during the 1920s; the latter is the more traditional, neo-Freudian position. Both view individuals as being driven from normal heterosexuality to homosexuality by the intrusion of fear arising from unconscious phantasies of imagined danger and conflict (Ovesey & Woods, 1980). It is not my purpose here to explain the origins of homosexuality that result from preoedipal or oedipal conflicts (for an excellent overview see Lewes, 1988), but to note how these two points of origin give rise to images of the self. The focus here is the sense of self-worth among those truly homosexual and not those who engage in homosexual behavior for what are assumed to be "situational reasons," such as not having heterosexual outlets while in detention centers or boarding schools (Brown, 1957).

Preoedipal Origins

During the preoedipal phase, usually before age 3 years, an individual attempts to resolve conflicts inherent in the separation anxiety that originates in the infantile desire to merge with the mother. Symbiotic fusion with the mother would allay this anxiety, but it would also provoke fears of engulfment and annihilation (Ovesey & Woods, 1980; Socarides, 1968). In the absence of any figure with whom to unite, the individual turns inward to the self, which results in excessive self-love (narcissism) and developmental arrest or ego deformity. For such an individual, life is a never-ending search for the sexual possession of a same-sex mate exactly like the self (Hatterer, 1970). This homosexual resolution manifests itself in the neurotic individual who has an inflated sense of self and what it means to be a man or a woman. It represents a regression to primordial instincts of self-centeredness (Stekel, 1922).

Thus, although the preoedipal homosexual narcissist may appear to have a positive self-image, glorifying the self with praise, fine clothing, and self-display, in actuality he or she suffers from an acute sense of inferiority and self-hatred (West, 1967). The alternative to the narcissistic state is a return to the amorphous, undifferentiated ego state of infancy, but any sense of individuality as a separate entity would be destroyed by such a regression (Socarides, 1968). Homosexuals are thus portrayed by these psychoanalysts as in need of punishment and self-damaging behavior; their sense of inferiority and guilt is viewed as reflecting deeply rooted shame, humiliation, and infantile fears. As noted by Socarides (1968), their pseudoconfidence and self-aggrandizement are only a facade for the reality of their intense and pervasive self-hatred.

Oedipal Origins

The second and later point of origin for homosexual development involves an unsuccessful resolution of oedipal conflicts that results in cross-sex identification and hence, by implication, same-sex sexual behavior. The homosexual girl does not, however, lose her feminine inferiority complex; in fact, it intensifies because she becomes both a "defective woman and an incomplete man." She resents her femininity, but realizes that she lacks the equipment necessary to seduce women that her male rivals possess (de Beauvoir, 1963). Unlike her heterosexual female peers, she is neither able nor willing to sublimate her feminine inferiority in order to form a gratifying, successful psychosexual relationship as a wife; to adequately run a home; and to bear and rear children. These are conditions that would boost her self-esteem (Romm, 1965). Rejected by her parents and others as unfeminine, the lesbian feels unloved, depreciated, and demeaned. Her depression and self-destructive behavior reflect her basic masochism. The sense of inferiority, demanded by her punitive superego, must be reversed in order to raise ego strength and self-esteem (Romm, 1965). The sorry state of the homosexual female includes jealousy, sadomasochism, hostility, self-pity, ambivalence, guilt feelings, and insecurity. Although not all lesbians are the same (some are not "butch"), there are common denominators: "Lesbians are basically unhappy people. Many admit their unhappiness but others are deceived by their pseudoadjustment to life. . . . In general their attitude toward themselves is a negative one" (Caprio, 1954, p. 180).

For the boy, severe parental discipline during the oedipal period undermines his capacity to assert his masculinity. Fantasized and feared punishments include castration and death if heterosexual contact is initiated (Kwawer, 1980). This loss of the masculine role impairs his self-image, resulting in depreciated self-confidence in both sexual and nonsexual activities. He lacks masculine competitiveness, has an intensified regressive dependency need, and passively surrenders to a feminine identification (Kwawer, 1980; Ovesey, 1965; Ovesey & Woods, 1980). The sorry state of the homosexual male includes emotional disturbance, fear of the other sex, feelings of inadequacy, self-destructive drives, self-abnegation, and compulsive desires.

Kaplan (1967, p. 358) also linked homosexuality with deficits in self-image: "The homosexual, however, is unable to love himself as he is, since he is too dissatisfied with himself; instead he loves his ego-ideal, as represented by the homosexual partner whom he chooses." Motivations to search for an ego ideal during the oedipal period arise in part from physical, social, and intellectual disturbances in self-image. These stem from preoedipal experiences and relationships that occur prior to the identification process. Thus, low self-esteem leads to homosexuality, at least in some instances.

Bridging Gaps

From a psychoanalytic perspective the homosexual is often portrayed as possessing self-hatred and a negative self-image. If the point of origin is preoedipal the homosexual individual will appear to be filled with self-love and to feel, at least on a conscious level, high self-esteem. But these are only superficial because they reflect a far deeper sense of inferiority. If the point of origin is oedipal, then everything the sexual invert feels and does mirrors his or her self-loathing.

Recently, there has been a concerted effort to bridge the antagonistic gap that frequently separates psychoanalytic theorists/therapists and the gay and lesbian communities. The perception of many gay males and lesbians is that, by definition, psychoanalysis views homosexual individuals as pathological and in need of corrective therapy (Cornett & Hudson, 1985; Hencken, 1982). The reconciliation between the two factions has involved minimizing the "contributions" of several anti-gay, post-Freudian theorists (e.g., Bieber and Socarides) and emphasizing a more holistic and Freudian view of psychoanalysis (Lewes, 1988). Psychotherapy can then be viewed as an aid in understanding and helping individuals who are in emotional pain. This approach can thus focus on a person's unique needs, desires, and history such that internal conflicts are relieved and control over one's life is maintained, regardless of sexual orientation (Cornett & Hudson, 1985). The goal is self-understanding and expression without assumptions or judgments regarding the pathology or nonpathology of sexual orientations (Herron, Kinter, Sollinger, & Trubowitz (1981/1982). This view is consistent, even inherent in the psychoanalytic method.

In describing the historical development of the antipathy between psychoanalysis and the gay and lesbian communities, Hencken (1982) noted that psychoanalysis is not a set of agreed-upon, monolithic visions of homosexuality. Thus, there are both pro- and anti-gay psychoanalytic theorists and concepts. Psychoanalysis has the capacity to increase our understanding of the historical meanings, motivations, and interpretations of homosexual behavior and homosexuality. Rather than emphasize the pathological nature of homosexuality, psychoanalysis should and can affirm and celebrate homosexuality.

SOCIOLOGICAL PERSPECTIVES

Sociological theorists are seldom concerned with classical psychological processes in linking the development of self-image with sexual orientation. Social labeling and symbolic interactionist approaches do not usually regard homosexuality as inherently pathological or deviant (Hammersmith, 1987). Rather, they emphasize the state of the external world and its subsequent impact on an individual's self-evaluation. Negative social definitions of one's identity, Weinberg (1983) wrote, will "cause feelings of guilt and self-hatred and attempts to reject the label. If an individual learns to view homosexuals negatively, guilt, fear, and ambivalence will accompany self-labeling as homosexual" (p. 36). Many have written on various aspects of a North American culture, frequently labeled homophobic, that influence the homosexual person to develop propensities for self-hatred.

In the 1950s Donald Webster Cory (a pseudonym) noted that psychological therapy, intended to help a homosexual become a well-integrated, happy invert, was frequently impeded by social conditions that were beyond the control of the therapist. The goal of therapy should be the enhancement of self-acceptance in the face of societal rejection. Cory (1951) warned that the "happy homosexual" must not accept social values imposed on him:

> They accept, with heads bowed—angry, hurt, and helpless—and often with some sense that perhaps their lot is not entirely without justification. . . . The worst effect of discrimination has been to make the homosexuals doubt themselves and share in the general contempt for sexual inverts. (p. 39)

The destructive nature and the guilt feelings characteristic of most "inverts" simply reflect an all too willing acceptance of the contempt that North American society has for most minorities.

This view was echoed in the 1960s in Magee's (1966) analysis of the homosexual's sense of guilt, shamefulness, and self-abasement that emanate from a subconscious acceptance of the majority's standards. In Hoffman's (1968) revelations of the gay world, a male homosexual's low self-esteem is attributed to the process of internalizing homophobic values and attitudes through the reflected appraisals of significant others in his world, especially those of parents, siblings, and teachers. Heterosexuality is encouraged and homosexuality is discouraged; one is natural and the other, unnatural. This is the message given to the child and to the adolescent. The homosexual individual's self-esteem will suffer as a result.

By the 1970s there was growing doubt among some as to the direct connection between societal attitudes and an individual's self-esteem. Dank (1971) noted that although a homosexual individual may know that he is deviant from a societal point of view, he often does not accept this judgment as his identity. The longer he is out the more likely he is to accept himself and deny society's evaluation of him as a bad person. Tripp (1975) also suggested that the more committed a man is to homosexuality the more likely he is to evolve adaptive mechanisms to protect the self against social rejection. To survive, the gay man often develops an even higher level of coping skills and self-regard than the average individual (Gagnon & Simon, 1973). Sociologists Sagarin and Kelly (1980, p. 372) noted that "the hostile societal reactions forces large numbers of deviants into a subcultural milieu of their own, where they give one another mutual support and an ideology that enhances the ego and the self-image."

An individual does not necessarily need to experience the negative social reaction directly. Sometimes the imagined fear of a negative sanction is more powerful than an actual assault on an individual's self-image. Through the mass media anti-homosexual cultural meanings and expectations are conveyed to the gay person. Indeed, Weinberg and Williams (1974) found that gay males who anticipated discrimination and believed that heterosexuals viewed them negatively had the lowest self-assessment.

Coleman (1982), a therapist, accepted the causal connection between negative societal views and negative conceptions of self as deviant, sick, or immoral. But many lesbians and gay men, even those in therapy, develop positive views of themselves through the counter efforts of family, friends, ministers, teachers, and counselors.

Others in the 1970s and 1980s (D'Emilio, 1983; Fox, 1983; Malyon, 1981; Nungesser, 1983; Ogg, 1978; Paul, 1982; Pennington, 1983; Saghir & Robins, 1980; Weinberg, 1983) noted the personal consequences of internalizing external attitudes and values. For example, Weinberg (1983, p. 244) stated, "The way people feel about themselves intimately relates to the kinds of feedback that they perceive they are getting from others." Several, however, reported exceptions. Saghir and Robins (1980) proposed that because female homosexuality is less stigmatized than male homosexuality in our culture, a lesbian has less internal conflict, turmoil, and subjective unhappiness. Paul (1982) believed that the new generation of young lesbians and gay males may not be as susceptible to a hostile society and thus are more likely to become healthy, high self-esteem individuals. Altman (1982) referred to these individuals as "the new homosexuals," who have a sense of community and the support offered by community organizations and activities, and who have rejected conventional heterosexual models. Although Rofes (1984) found support for this view in terms of sexuality, gender distinctions, and politics, lesbian and gay youth still feel isolated and in need of support in their homes, neighborhoods, and schools. This is because, Nungesser (1983) noted, many in our culture initially accept the beliefs and fears of homosexual acts, actors, and life-styles. On the basis of the view that the self-concept is an internalized representation of social norms and beliefs, a youth's self-esteem will suffer if a homosexual identity is salient in the total image of the self.

Few of these writers have been explicit about the process by which the external becomes internalized. Rather, the connection is more correlational conceptually—that is, the external and the internal occur together. Social oppression, stigma, and an internalized self-hatred in gay people are somehow related. D'Emilio (1983) was most explicit,

> The condemnations that did occur burdened homosexuals and lesbians with a corrosive self-image. The dominant view of them—as perverts, psychopaths, deviates, and the like—seeped into their consciousness. Shunted to the margins of American society, harassed because of their sexuality, many gay men and women internalized the negative descriptions and came to embody the stereotypes. . . . Whether seen from the vantage point of religion, medicine, or the law, the homosexual or lesbian was a flawed individual, not a victim of injustice. (p. 53)

Other historians (Boswell, 1980; Bullough, 1976; Katz, 1976) have also speculated that governments and religions contributed heavily to a negative portrait of homosexuality. Fox (1983) referred to the present-day church as "homophobic," handicapping the spiritual growth of gay men and lesbians. The result is psycho-spiritual arrest and a broken, lonely person. Self-affirmation and self-acceptance are thus difficult for the gay or lesbian Christian who is constantly reminded that being homosexual is sinful (Pennington, 1983).

Hencken (1982) proposed that as researchers we need to study the development of the psychological processes that occur under negative social attitudes (the inter-nalization of oppression). He noted, "We know a good deal about the external conditions of oppression and about some of its consequences, but between the causes and the effects live individual human beings" (p. 138).

EMPIRICAL RESEARCH

Hooker concluded from her simple but revolutionary research with a non-clinically-based homosexual sample (1957, 1963, 1965) that as a clinical entity homosexuality does not exist. There are many forms with just as many outcomes. Thus, to assert that homosexual persons are necessarily maladjusted individuals filled with self-loathing and low self-esteem is a generalization without empirical support from her projective study of male homosexuals. If, in fact, some homosex-uals have a negative attitude toward the self, then it is an empirical question as to whether it is inherent in the personality structure of the individual (psychoanalysis) or the result of victimization from a hostile world (sociological theory) (Hooker, 1965).

Reviewers of literature on the psychological adjustment of gay men and lesbi-ans (e.g., Gonsiorek, 1977; Hart et al., 1978) concluded that there are no essential mental health consequences of sexual orientation. One dimension of psychological adjustment, self-esteem, has received substantial empirical investigation. Differen-tiated by sex, the following studies address the theoretical assumption that being homosexual and hating oneself cohabitate. They are not all equal in methodologi-cal or design rigor, and this issue will be discussed in a later section.

Females

Empirical studies generally report either relatively few differences in self-esteem level among women of different sexual orientations or higher scores among lesbians. For example, an early study by Saghir and Robins (1973) reported the same level (20%) of low self-esteem and self-confidence among lesbian volunteers in the Chicago and San Francisco chapters of the sociopolitical organization Daughters of Bilitis and heterosexual women recruited from St. Louis apartment residents. Self-esteem was assessed by a structured interview. Table 2.1 summa-rizes the 16 published studies I found that compared aspects of self-concept among lesbians and groups of heterosexual women. Eight reported no difference, six scored lesbians higher, and two reported higher self-esteem for heterosexuals.

Lesbians from New York City and London had higher self-acceptance scores on the Dignan Scale of Self-Acceptance than "matched" heterosexual women (Siegelman, 1972a, 1979). The lesbians completing the questionnaires were re-cruited from political groups (Daughters of Bilitis), feminist organizations, ho-mophile bookstores, and newspaper advertisements. As a group they were highly

Table 2.1 Studies comparing the self-concept of lesbian and heterosexual women

Year	Authors	N	Lesbians Sample	Measure	Results
1968, 1971	Freedman	81	New York Daughters of Bilitis	Personal Orientation Inventory	No difference in self-acceptance
1969	Hopkins	24	Research volunteers	Cattell's 16 Personality Factor Questionnaire	Lesbians more self-sufficient
1971	Thompson, McCandless, and Strickland	84	Friendship networks	Adjective Check List and Semantic Differential	Lesbians higher in self-confidence
1971	Wilson and Greene	50	Friends (Denver)	California Psychological Inventory	No difference in self-acceptance and sense of well-being
1972a	Siegelman	84	Daughters of Bilitis, bookstore	Dignan Scale of Self-Acceptance	Lesbians higher in self-acceptance
1973	Saghir and Robins	61	San Francisco and Chicago Daughters of Bilitis	Interview	No difference in self-esteem and self-confidence
1974	Ohlson and Wilson	64	Gay Liberation Front (Denver)	Minnesota Multiphasic Personality Inventory	Lesbians more secure and self-confident
1976	Greenberg	8	Mattachine Society (Buffalo)	Rosenberg Self-Esteem Scale	No difference in self-esteem
1978, 1981	Bell and Weinberg; Bell, Weinberg, and Hammersmith	229	Advertisements, bars, personal contacts, organizations, mailing lists, and public places (San Francisco)	Rosenberg Self-Esteem Scale	Lesbians lower in self-esteem; close-coupleds, functionals, and asexual lesbians equal in self-esteem to straight women
1979	Dailey	5	Volunteer couples	Hudson Index of Self-Esteem	Lesbians lowest in self-esteem
1979	Siegelman	61	Lesbian organizations (London)	Dignan Scale of Self-Acceptance	Lesbians higher in self-acceptance
1979	Strassberg, Roback, Cunningham, McKee, and Larson	40	Campus and church groups	Tennessee Self-Concept Scale	No difference in self-concept
1979	Weis and Dain	50	Students from university organizations and classes, friendship networks, public places	Loevinger's ego stages	No difference in ego level
1981	Larson	40	Self-consciousness groups	Tennessee Self-Concept Scale	Lesbians higher in self-satisfaction
1983	La Torre and Wendenburg	18 lesbian, 2 bisexual	Women's Center and undergraduates	Rosenberg Self-Esteem Scale	No difference in self-esteem
1985	Mervis	30	Friends	Rorschach	No difference in self-confidence

educated, professional women in their 30s. Few were ever in therapy; they were highly goal directed and scored low on depression.

In another study (LaTorre & Wendenburg, 1983), 125 volunteers from a British Columbia women's center and four psychology courses completed a four-page questionnaire. Two groups of women, self-labeled lesbians and women who said they preferred sex with other women, did not differ in their Rosenberg Self-Esteem Scale scores from four other groups of women: heterosexuals, bisexuals, those who preferred sex with men, and those who had no preference. The numbers in the first two categories, however, were quite small (18 and 20, respectively).

On the whole, the studies summarized in Table 2.1 were conducted primarily with lesbians who were White, well educated, politically active, vocationally skilled, and young. The research strategies and findings of Bell and Weinberg (1978; Bell, Weinberg, & Hammersmith, 1981a, 1981b) differ from the above. They recruited a large sample of lesbians in San Francisco (which they do not claim is a representative population of lesbians). A cross-section subsample of these women, representing a range of ages, religions, social classes, educational levels, and residential variables, was selected for intensive study. The lesbians scored lower than matched straight women on the Rosenberg Self-Esteem Scale. Few of the lesbians recalled a happy adolescence; many felt anxious, inadequate, and negative during the adolescent years. These variables did not, however, predict whether a girl would become a heterosexual or homosexual adult.

Males

Empirical studies that compare male sexual orientation groups are far more plentiful than the research summarized above on women. These studies generally find relatively few differences between homosexual and heterosexual males in feelings of self-worth and self-acceptance (see Table 2.2). Gay men in general felt good about their lives. Spada (1979) received 1,038 responses from 10,000 questionnaires that were distributed in gay bars, meetings, bookstores, and magazines. Only 13% said they were not happy. Among gay male couples interviewed, 68% described their childhood as happy or harmonious (McWhirter & Mattison, 1984). These men were between the ages of 20 and 69 years and were recommended for participation by previous research subjects. Saghir and Robins (1973) studied 104 men in homophile organizations and friends of members. Although more homosexual than heterosexual men reported generally poor confidence and self-esteem, the difference was not significant. The vast majority of both groups maintained adequate levels of self-confidence and self-esteem.

Green's (1987) clinical samples of 35 "feminine" (primarily gay) and 26 "masculine" (primarily straight) adolescent and young adult males did not differ on a self-concept measure assessing moral ethical self (feelings of being a good or bad person), family self, social self, general maladjustment, and personality integration. The former scored lower, however, on self-satisfaction (self-acceptance), physical self, and personal self. But within this feminine group there were no differences in self-concept scores among those who evolved into homosexual or bisexual adults and those who became heterosexual.

Several studies, many suspect because of methodological or sampling shortcomings, report gay males to be deficient in self-worth. For example, predomi-

Table 2.2 Studies comparing the self-concept of gay and heterosexual men

Year	Authors	N	Sample	Measure	Results
			Gay men		
1960	Chang and Block	20	Friendship networks	A real and ideal adjective checklist	No difference in self-acceptance
1960	Doidge and Holtzman	20	"Gay" Air Force psychiatric clinic	Minnesota Multiphasic Personality Inventory	Gays lower in self-confidence
1962	Cattell and Morony	100	Prisoners convicted homosexual acts (Australian) Unconvicted (Australian)	Cattell's 16 Personality Factor Questionnaire	No difference in self-sufficiency
1962	Bieber et al.	106	Treatment patients	Treatment interview	Gays lower in childhood feelings
1964	Dean and Richardson	40	Overt gays	Minnesota Multiphasic Personality Inventory	No difference in self-confidence
1970	Evans	44	Gay organizations (Los Angeles)	Cattell's 16 Personality Factor Questionnaire	Gays higher in self-sufficiency
1971	Evans	44	Gay organizations (Los Angeles)	Adjective Check List	Gays lower in self-confidence
1971	Thompson, McCandless, and Strickland	127	Friendship networks	Adjective Check List and Semantic Differential	No difference in self-concept, gays lower in self-confidence
1972b	Siegelman	307	Homophile organizations, friendship networks, public places	Dignan Scale of Self-Acceptance	Gays higher in self-acceptance
1973	Greenberg	89	Gay organizations	RSE[a]	No difference in self-esteem
1973	Saghir and Robins	84	Homophile organizations (San Francisco and Chicago)	Interview	No difference in self-esteem and self-confidence
1974b	Myrick	276	Bar patrons (Texas)	RSE[a], questionnaire	Gays lower in self-esteem and self-acceptance
1974	Weinberg and Williams	1,057 (US), 1,064 (Netherlands), 252 (Denmark)	Gay clubs, bars, and organizations	Questionnaire, RSE[a]	No difference in self-esteem
1976	Greenberg	11	Mattachine Society (Buffalo)	RSE[a]	No difference in self-esteem
1978, 1981	Bell and Weinberg; Bell, Weinberg, and Hammersmith	575	Advertisements, bars, personal contacts, baths, organizations, mailing lists, and public places (San Francisco)	RSE[a]	Gays lower in self-esteem; functionals and close-coupled gays equal in self-esteem to straight men
1978	Siegelman	84	Advertisements and gay organizations (London)	Dignan Scale of Self-Acceptance	No difference in self-acceptance
1979	Dailey	5	Volunteer couples	Hudson Index of Self-Esteem	No difference in self-esteem

(Table continues on next page)

21

Table 2.2 Studies comparing the self-concept of gay and heterosexual men (*Continued*)

Year	Authors				
		Gay men			
		N	Sample	Measure	Results
1979	Hooberman	37	Newspaper advertisements (University of Michigan)	RSE[a]	No difference in self-esteem
1979	Prytula, Wellford, and DeMonbreun	28	Friendship networks	Questionnaire	Gays lower in recall of childhood self-concept
1979	Spada	1,038	National survey	Questionnaire	Most gays said "happy"
1979	Weis and Dain	50	Students from friendship networks, public places, university classes, and organizations	Loevinger's ego stages	No difference in ego level
1981	Larson	40	Self-consciousness groups	TSCS[b]	No difference in self-satisfaction
1981	Skrapec and MacKenzie	8	Volunteers	RSE[a]	Gays highest in self-esteem
1982	Berger	112	Advertisements and recruitments	Modified RSE[a] and life satisfaction scale	Gays higher in life satisfaction and self-acceptance
1983	Harry	1,556	Newspaper advertisements (Chicago)	Questionnaire	No difference in self-acceptance
1983	Mallen	30	Homophile and activist groups, friendship networks, church group (Australian)	Questionnaire	No difference in real/ideal self-distance
1984	Lutz, Roback, and Hart	65	Volunteers, church group	TSCS[b]	No difference in self-concept
1984	McWhirter and Mattison	156	Couples, friendship networks (San Diego)	Interview	Most said happy childhood
1985	Wayson	58	Business and professional groups	Test of Attentional and Interpersonal Style	No difference in self-esteem
1987	Green	35	Treatment clients	TSCS[b]	No difference in self-concept; gays lower in self-acceptance

[a]Rosenberg Self-Esteem Scale.
[b]Tennessee Self-Concept Scale.

nantly homosexual men referred (apparently arrested for sexual offenses) to a psychiatric clinic at an Air Force base in the 1950s had lower self-confidence scores than "normal" and disciplined heterosexuals and predominantly heterosexuals with some homosexual experience (Doidge & Holtzman, 1960). An often cited study by Bieber et al. (1962) surveyed therapists who were treating homosexual clients. The 106 cases of homosexual males that were submitted were more likely than 100 straight men in therapy to report that as a child they had negative feelings (lone wolf, frail, clumsy) about themselves.

Several studies, not any more representative of gay men than the previously cited research, found higher self-acceptance levels among homosexual than heterosexual men. In a sample of 112 males over 40 years old, Berger (1982) reported that 82% scored high on self-acceptance; 84% reported feeling very or pretty happy; and 85% responded "never" or "infrequent" to the question, "Does knowing you're gay weigh on your mind and make you feel guilty, depressed, anxious, or ashamed?" The sample mean of 74.5 on life satisfaction was higher than most reports based on samples of heterosexuals. Siegelman (1972b) found gay men to have higher levels of self-acceptance than a group of undergraduate and graduate male students at a New York City university. The 307 gay men were recruited from the Mattachine Society of New York, homophile bookstore announcements, lectures on homosexuality, and gay friends. These findings were replicated with a group of 84 London gay men (Siegelman, 1978).

Two studies that sampled a wider cross-section of gay males than the above research provide divergent results. Gays scored lower than a matched straight sample on the Rosenberg Self-Esteem Scale (Bell & Weinberg, 1978) and were more likely to recall feeling unhappy, inadequate, anxious, and negative about the self while growing up (Bell et al., 1981a, 1981b). But this view of the self as a child was inconsequential for the development of sexual orientation; neither was it descriptive of gay males who were characterized as functionals ("swinging singles") or close-coupleds ("happily marrieds") (Bell & Weinberg, 1978).

In the second study (Weinberg & Williams, 1974), a 145-item questionnaire was given or mailed to gay males living in New York, San Francisco, Amsterdam, and Copenhagen at clubs, bars, and homophile organizations. The sample consisted of 1,057 gay males from the United States; 1,064 from the Netherlands; and 252 from Denmark. Overall, the men were somewhat overrepresentative of the urban, young, highly educated, and well-to-do gay. They did not differ in self-esteem from a sample drawn randomly from telephone books.

Conclusion

Although many studies concluded there was no difference in the self-esteem of homosexual and heterosexual women, almost as many reported that lesbians had a higher level of self-evaluation than groups of heterosexuals. Of the 30 studies of men reviewed, 17 found few differences in global self-evaluation between gay and straight men. In six studies gay males had lower self-acceptance than did straight men, four found the reverse, and three were indeterminable. It is difficult to compare these studies given the diversity of populations sampled and measures used, but it would appear that Greenberg's (1973, pp. 141–142) conclusion is warranted: "Though feeling alienated from the society in which they lived, [homosexuals] were satisfied with their homosexuality to the extent that they exhibited self-esteem scores that were comparable to heterosexual scores obtained on the same instrument."

The approach of Bell and Weinberg (1978) to categorize lesbians and gay men on the basis of sexual experiences, personality attributes, and social conditions would appear to be a superior approach. For example, three of their "types" of lesbians were equal in self-esteem to heterosexual women: Close-coupleds ("happily marrieds"), functionals ("swinging singles"), and asexuals ("loners"). Perhaps a similar division of straight women or of straight men would also reveal self-esteem differences, creating self-esteem groupings within the heterosexual population. This is an important study because of its focus on intra-gay rather than straight/gay differences. This will be considered in greater detail in subsequent chapters.

MEANINGS AND CONJECTURES

The Theories

Sagarin and Kelly (1980) argued that one's theoretical bias can become a blinder: "People seem to have begun with their conclusion, and then utilized that portion of the evidence at hand to fortify such a conclusion, rather than the reverse" (p. 366). For example, DuMas's (1979) "review" of the self-evaluation literature found a "number of studies" showing homosexuals to have low self-esteem. His citations included only publications by psychoanalytically oriented writers. The title of his book, *Gay Is Not Good*, hints at his moral perspective as well.

The burden of proof is on those theorists, in both the psychoanalytic and sociological fields, who charge that homosexual persons are maladjusted and psychologically unhealthy to produce acceptable empirical justification. Clinical psychologists and psychiatrists frequently present their patients as sufficient proof but many have critiqued their methodologies and findings (Churchill, 1967; Fluckiger, 1966; Lewes, 1988; Weinberg, 1972). Very little is illustrated by such data aside from exemplifying how to confirm what one has already affirmed. D. Sanders (1980) noted several problems underlying the psychoanalytic approach. Frequently, the homosexual label is applied equally to those who have had a single adolescent instance and those who have made a lifelong commitment. Not all homosexuals are the same, either in life-style or etiology. Sanders also doubted the assumption that sexual behavior causes personality difficulties. In reality the two may be only correlated, or not correlated at all. Finally, the homosexual population for most psychiatrists consists only of patients who come for help. He challenged psychiatrists to separate psychological problems from sexual orientation: Treat the low self-esteem and do not attempt to cure the sexual orientation.

Thus, psychoanalysis is suspect in the eyes of many because of its moralism, a stance that is somewhat surprising given Freud's more humane approach (Lewes, 1988). Freud (1962) believed that multiple types of homosexuality existed, that homosexuals are not sick, and that many homosexuals are apparently "normal" if not exceptional in all other ways. There is no vice, or anything to be ashamed about, in homosexuality. He noted, "Psychoanalytic research very strongly opposes the attempt to separate homosexuals from other persons as a group of a special natural" (p. 10). Psychiatrists more moderate than Bieber and more neo-Freudian agree. For example, Kirkpatrick and Morgan (1980) maintained that homosexuality by itself is not an indicator of poor psychological functioning. Many lesbians and gay males adapt to a hostile environment with little or no deleterious consequences for self-evaluation or for leading a loving and productive life. I believe Freud would agree.

Sociological theorists rely on more "scientific" empirical studies to substantiate their theoretical position that gay men and lesbians have low self-esteem. But these studies are also frequently and woefully inadequate and contradictory. Social theorists assume, without empirical evidence, that a homophobic society is instrumental in creating self-hatred among gay men and lesbians. For example, D'Emilio (1983) wrote,

> But anti-homosexualism prevaded American culture, and it infected the consciousness of gay men and women no less than heterosexuals. Homosexuals and lesbians absorbed views of themselves as immoral, depraved, and pathological individuals; many accepted harassment and punishment as well deserved. (p. 124)

Yet, as evident from the empirical research reviewed in this chapter, it has not been demonstrated that gay males and lesbians have a deficient self-acceptance level. I affirm that in the United States gay men and lesbians have grown up in a homophobic culture, and I do not deny that this hatred has consequences. But to my knowledge, the causal link between the external hatred and the internal self-loathing has not been established; nor has it been documented that the two are highly correlated with each other, that is, that gay males and lesbians growing up in a homophobic society have lower self-esteem than those reared in a less homophobic society. This should not be particularly surprising because few researchers have provided data demonstrating that self-esteem is caused by or significantly correlated with large-scale sociostructural variables (Savin-Williams & Demo, 1983a).

Thus, although lesbians and gay men may recognize that their sexual behavior is deviant by cultural norms, it is not necessary to generalize this "deviance" to other aspects of the self. We too can compartmentalize aspects of our lives and adapt (Weinberg & Williams, 1974). Vining (1988) chastised gay writers, especially social historians, for taking the "gay" out of our history. He maintained that our elders survived with "lifetimes of great happiness, lives full of fondly remembered sexual experiences and happy matings—despite the restrictions the law tried to impose against both" (p. 9). Although I am sure that this was not a universal experience or perspective, nevertheless professionals may have lost contact with and thus distorted the lives of the gay male and lesbian rank and file by emphasizing the negative in our history and culture. We may have lost sight of our resiliency and our joy.

Research Design

It would not be terribly difficult to discredit on grounds of inadequacies the research designs, procedures, or samples of many of the studies reviewed in this chapter. Bell (1975) and Weinberg (Weinberg & Bell, 1972) questioned more generally the research designs and methodological procedures of most studies of homosexuality. Samples are usually small and drawn from a biased subset of the total lesbian and gay population; instruments are frequently subjectively constructed, administered, and evaluated; gays and straights are assumed to constitute a simple dichotomy; and heterosexual and homosexual samples are rarely adequately matched. The manner in which most research studies define the sexual orientation of their subjects has been seriously and convincingly challenged (Coleman, 1987; Klein, Sepekoff, & Wolf, 1985; Shively & DeCecco, 1977; Suppe, 1984).

Although studies of lesbian and gay male self-esteem are usually based on a small sample size, there are notable exceptions (Bell & Weinberg, 1978; Harry, 1983; Siegelman, 1972a, 1972b; Spada, 1979; Weinberg & Williams, 1974). Through many time-consuming and innovative techniques, Bell and Weinberg (Bell & Weinberg, 1978; Bell et al., 1981a, 1981b) recruited research participants from bars, social clubs, political organizations, baths, friendship networks, and advertisements. These large studies are still not able to draw a representative sample of gay males and lesbians. They usually miss those most fearful, bisexuals, ethnic minorities, married lesbians and gay men, those who do not volunteer for research projects, those not publicly out, and those living in nonurban settings. But as men and women become increasingly comfortable expressing and affirming their sexual orientation, they become more accessible as research participants. Thus, present-day investigators of self-evaluation have an advantage not afforded earlier psychologists and sociologists: a larger and more representative sample of the lesbian and gay population.

Another issue that is only sparingly addressed is the diversity within the gay and lesbian population. Weinberg and Williams (1974) extensively documented this diversity by noting how such variables as age, social class, sex role, subjective assessments of being out and discriminated against, living arrangements, religious feelings, and social involvement influence psychological adjustment. Categorizing gay males and lesbians by profiles based on personality and social behavior was exceedingly useful for Bell and Weinberg (1978) in understanding variability on self-evaluation. "Functionals" and "close-coupleds" of both sexes had higher self-acceptance levels than the other subgroups. The reasons for this were not given. Commitment to others (Hammersmith & Weinberg, 1973) explains the latter but not the former group. Few studies have untangled the mystery of why some gay men and lesbians have higher self-esteem than others.

One of the primary research issues that Bell et al. (1981a) explored was whether becoming homosexual is linked with level of self-acceptance. They suggested, as others have (e.g., Saghir & Robins, 1973), that homosexuality has many causes and assumes many forms of expression. Reinforcing this diversity, Kirkpatrick and Morgan (1980) linked self-evaluation level with the purpose that homosexuality has for the individual. For example, they asserted that female homosexual behavior may be a developmental phase related to consolidation of a feminine identity, a regression from the anxieties of the oedipal period, a preoedipal gender disorder with specific narcissistic defects, or a temporary adaptation to a bad relationship or when heterosexual pairing is not possible. Self-evaluation level among lesbians will vary as a function of the relevance of these patterns. Berger (1982) believed that those who are most integrated into the gay community, who are not concerned with concealing or changing their sexual orientation, and who find support through relationships and friendships have the highest levels of self-esteem. It is difficult, however, to separate cause from effect. High self-esteem may be a result of these factors, or perhaps one with already positive self-esteem becomes involved with others, is not concerned with passing, and joins social and political groups. We have few leads in these matters.

To assume that lesbians and gay men form a homogeneous class of people belittles and reduces individuals to sexual beings. Sexuality is one aspect of a daily life, but it is not the totality. Research has traditionally contrasted homosexual and heterosexual individuals; occasionally bisexuals were added to the comparisons. Very early, West (1967, p. 48) noted, "Generalizations about homosexual temperament are no safer than generalizations about homosexual physique." Yet, the generalizations continued and new paradigms, in which comparisons are made within the lesbian and gay population, remain unfulfilled.

It is also important not to generalize from studies of gay males to lesbians. Female homosexuality is a uniquely female phenomenon and is neither the same nor the inverse of male homosexuality (Kirkpatrick & Morgan, 1980; Ponse, 1980; Richardson, 1981a, 1981b). For example, Weinberg (1972) attributed the high self-esteem of lesbians to the fact that the process of internalizing cultural homophobia is not as strong among lesbians because girls are not as forcibly instructed to shun boyishness as boys are instructed to avoid girlishness. Thus, sexism—there is nothing worse for the growing boy than being effeminate!—may be as involved as homophobia in accounting for variations among gay males and lesbians in self-evaluation. Psychoanalytic theory also explains this gender difference. Because the object choice of females is flexible and their need for intimacy with another female is a natural part of their emotional life, a homosexual affair is less threatening to their sense of self and self-evaluation (Kirkpatrick & Morgan, 1980). In fact, self-esteem may be restored with a loving, intimate relationship with a woman. Gender differences in self-esteem, coming out, and the relations of various factors with these two are addressed in later chapters of this book.

CONCLUSION

The "puzzling normality of the well-adjusted homosexual," noted by West (1967, p. 265), is not easily explained by either psychoanalytic or sociological theory but is nevertheless well documented by empirical research reviewed in this chapter. Self-evaluation among gay men and lesbians is considered by many to be so fluid as to be easily altered by changes in the environment (joining a gay or lesbian organization) or in one's personal identity (coming out). West suggested, however, that self-concept is a crystallized characteristic and is heavily influenced by one's developmental history and temperament. These issues have not been adequately addressed in the literature on homosexuality. If this position is accurate, then self-esteem among gay men and lesbians is congruent with other personality variables, regardless of the sexual orientation of the population studied. Although it is probably of no advantage for one's self-assessment to live in a homophobic society or to have preoedipal or oedipal conflicts with one's parents, many gay men and lesbians adapt to survive with intact and healthy egos (D. Sanders, 1980).

Counter to this perspective is the oppressive view of homosexuality usually attributed to American psychiatrists, well represented by Bieber in a 1971 *Playboy* panel discussion. For Bieber, homosexuality is a psychologically rooted sexual disorder, similar to female frigidity and male impotence, that is based on neurotic fears of heterosexual inadequacy and a seriously impaired sense of masculinity/ femininity. In the same interview Dick Leitsch, a spokesperson for many gay causes, refuted Bieber's theory but not his conclusions. If gay men are psycho-pathological, paranoid, and criminal then it is because society so considers and treats gays. As a result, "You obviously develop feelings of being inadequate and unwanted" (*Playboy* panel, 1971, p. 70).

These theories must be challenged because neither is supported by research data. In addition, I question the research strategy of comparing homosexual with heterosexual individuals. Over a decade ago Sang (1978) called on her colleagues to move away from research that poses the question, "Who is healthier, gays or straights?" (p. 80). Far more profitable, from both theoretical and empirical per-spectives, is to examine self-esteem variations within lesbian and gay populations. This was suggested in reviews (Harry, 1983; Hart et al., 1978) of sex role orienta-tion among lesbians and gay men. One purpose of this research project is to extend this strategy beyond the issue of sex role orientation to include multiple ways in which gay males and lesbians might differ.

Many years after Bell (1975) discussed the research needs for the study of homosexuality we are still at the drawing board. Greenberg (1973) and Hart et al. (1978) concluded that evidence relative to the self-concept of gay men and lesbians is contradictory in nature and could be attributed to such extraneous factors as subject selection, the person's greater self-disclosure level, and normal range vari-ations among other possibilities. The present research project was designed and carried out to address some of these issues.

3

Coming Out

OVERVIEW

Until fairly recently it was generally assumed that almost all gay males and lesbians went to great lengths to keep their homosexuality a secret. Gay pride was a dream, moral value and mental stability an illusion. Several factors served to perpetuate this image of the secretive and closeted gay. The "gay liberation movement had yet begun to challenge heterosexuals' stereotypes of homosexual individuals, assault the behemoth of social discrimination, or urge gays to 'come out of the closets and into the streets' " to openly embrace a gay identity (Bell & Weinberg, 1978, p. 62). Few societal institutions came forth on their own to declare a moratorium on social and legal discrimination, to counter cultural stereotypes, and to overturn moral condemnation. Descriptions of gay men and lesbians in popular, clinical, and scientific publications implied that disclosure was accompanied by ridicule, censure, and violent attacks (Weinberg & Williams, 1974). Also, traditional Judeo-Christian sanctions against homosexuality caused many to hesitate before disclosing their sexual identity. Religion, at its best, offered only forgiveness. Antihomosexual laws which threatened exposure and incarceration reinforced negative evaluations of homosexuality among the general public and effectively scared many gay men and women from openly disclosing their identity.

Bell and Weinberg (1978) noted that a different image of homosexual candor emerged during the 1970s.

> Many churches have examined their traditional attitudes toward homosexuality, a growing number of states have decriminalized homosexual activities, well-known and highly regarded persons have publicly acknowledged their homosexuality, and the mass media have discussed these events dispassionately. (p. 63)

In addition, the gay liberation movement became a powerful, visible social and political force. Although these liberal processes suggest that lesbians and gay men can now safely and openly disclose their sexual identity, antihomosexual attitudes and behaviors are still prevalent. Consequently, many either do not disclose their sexual orientation to others or do so only to select others. Thus, despite the apparent emergence of a more accepting society, gay men and lesbians continue to differ among themselves in the extent to which they are willing to openly express their sexual identity (Bell & Weinberg, 1978).

My appreciation is extended to Dr. Rand Lenhart for assistance in writing portions of this chapter.

Various aspects are involved in the move from "in the closet" to self and others to "out of the closet":

> As a developmental process through which gay persons become aware of their affectional
> and sexual preferences and choose to integrate this knowledge into their personal and social
> lives, coming out involves adopting a nontraditional identity, restructuring one's self-concept,
> reorganizing one's personal sense of history, and altering one's relations with others and with
> society . . . all of which reflects a complex series of cognitive and affective transformations as
> well as changes in behavior. (McDonald, 1982, p. 47)

DEFINITIONS

The Issues

Disclosure of sexual orientation is of concern to researchers as well as to gay men and lesbians. Despite the importance attached to how out a person is, little is known concerning the coming-out process and the impact it has on the individual. The term "coming out" is frequently used to refer to the process of identifying oneself as gay, lesbian, or bisexual, and yet there is no consensual meaning of the term. Weinberg and Williams (1974) pointed out that both theoretical writings and empirical research emphasize the covert–overt, known-aboutness aspects of coming out. Coming out is considered to be an ongoing process that takes place before an ever-expanding "series of audiences" (Ponse, 1980). The variable coming out is frequently cited as the major obstacle to acquiring a representative sample of gay men and lesbians for research purposes (Bell, 1975; Warren, 1977) and as a crucial factor affecting sexual, psychological, and social functioning (Weinberg & Williams, 1974).

"Coming out" refers to a process during which a number of milestone events occur whereby an individual moves from nonrecognition of his or her homosexuality, with perhaps a degree of sensitization of being somehow different from others, to self-recognition that he or she is indeed a homosexual person. The first "audience" is usually the self (Ponse, 1980). Whether this process must also include explorations of the gay or lesbian community, revelations to significant and nonsignificant others of this discovery, and self-acceptance as well as self-acknowledgment of homosexuality in order to be legitimately categorized as coming out is a matter of some theoretical disagreement within the social science literature. There are no rules in the coming-out process (Ponse, 1980). Early coming-out definitions tended to emphasize the social side, disclosure to others. More modern versions frequently include the tripartite dimensions of the social historian D'Emilio (1983): recognition of same-sex desires, subsequent attempts to act on those desires and preferences, and acknowledgment of one's sexual orientation to others of the same persuasion. The missing link here, occasionally included by others, is publicly coming out to all who care to know, especially to heterosexuals.

Any attempt to delineate the complex process of coming out and its impact on dimensions of psychological adjustment must, by necessity, be in some sense arbitrary and certainly cautious. Despite the fact that many of the models reviewed present coming out as a homogeneous, steplike sequence, in reality it is a continuous process with many backward steps accompanying the forward ones made by an emerging gay male or lesbian. McDonald (1982) referred to coming out as an "arduous developmental process" that frequently extends into adulthood. Proceeding through the process may help or hinder personal growth and self-image, depending in large part on one's prior maturity (Nemeyer, 1980). Although occasionally fate or chance events influence the process, coming out also involves individually derived choices that affect one's emerging sense of self (McDonald, 1982). The most frequently reported reasons given for not coming out are a fear of the unknown; a desire not to hurt or disappoint a loved one(s), usually one's parents (Cramer, 1986); and an avoidance of being rejected by parents and peers (Rector, 1982). Among lesbian adults Fitzpatrick (1983) reported the major reasons for not disclosing were the desire not to hurt or disappoint the family, fear of job loss, and fear of rejection; the reports of gay males are essentially the same. The positive consequences of coming out include a sense of freedom, of being oneself, of not living a lie, and of experiencing genuine acceptance (Fitzpatrick, 1983).

Most coming-out models propose an orderly or linear series of developmental stages based on a particular theoretical perspective (e.g., Erikson, Freud, Piaget, or Goffman). The step after an initial sense of feeling different is an awareness of sexual attractions that feel natural to the individual but are alien to those experienced by many of the individual's peers. Self-recognition is the next step. At some point, once homosexual feelings have been initially accepted and integrated, the individual must confront the next developmental task, disclosure to others (Coleman, 1982). Malyon (1981) noted that being known as a lesbian or gay, whether that knowledge is under the individual's control in terms of who knows or whether the individual is generally out to anyone who cares to know, is an important developmental milestone in identity-formation for many gay and lesbian youth. The stakes are quite high: "The suppression of homosexual impulses during primary adolescence results in an interruption and mitigation of the process of identity formation. The coming-out experience prompts another phase of psychological growth, similar to that which has primacy during age-appropriate adolescence" (p. 329).

Sophie (1985/1986) reviewed six theories of gay identity development to determine their internal consistency and applicability for her exploratory study of 14 women. She found four essential stages of identity development with common characteristics:

1. First awareness
   • Initial cognitive and emotional realization that one is "different" and that homosexuality may be the relevant issue
     • No disclosure to others
     • A feeling of alienation from oneself and others
2. Testing and exploration
     • Testing must precede acceptance of one's homosexuality
     • Initial but limited contact with the gay and lesbian community or with individual gay males and lesbians (but no relationships)
       • Alienation from heterosexuals
3. Identity acceptance
     • Preference for social interactions with other gay males and lesbians
     • Negative identity gives way to a positive identity
     • Initial disclosure to heterosexuals
4. Identity integration

- Views self as gay or lesbian with accompanying anger and pride in the identity
  - Disclosure to many others; public coming out
  - Identity stability; individual is unwilling and unable to change

Sophie discovered that although her data fit the broad outlines of these stages, in the specifics there were many variations.

Broadly speaking, coming-out models can be divided into three types, based on whether the primary emphasis is on internal processes (usually termed "identity"), external manifestations (disclosure or overtness), or some combination of these two. The first and last types are briefly reviewed below. Disclosure to others, the definition of coming out I used in the research reported in this book, is discussed in detail in Chapter 7.

Identity of Self

Those who focus on the internal, identity aspects of coming out apply a model based on theorists such as Piaget, Erikson, or Freud which was developed in another context (e.g., to explain cognitive, psychosocial, or psychosexual processes) to trace the evolution of homosexuality within an individual. Few empirical investigators include such dimensions, probably because of the difficulty in delineating, measuring, and validating identity components of development (Smith, 1983). As one part of the identity process most theorists include a stage, usually at the midway point, when self-disclosure to others is a necessary developmental marker. The primary emphasis remains, however, with internal issues of self-recognition and acceptance. For example, some (e.g., Benitez, 1983) have examined how an individual comes to define the self as homosexual over time; others (e.g., Brady, 1985), how an individual progresses through the identity stages of tolerance, acceptance, pride, and synthesis.

Cass's theoretical model (1979, 1984) included the acquisition of a homosexual identity as a significant aspect of self for the gay or lesbian person. In this process one must consider how identity is influenced by interactions that occur between individuals and the environment (Cass, 1979). Identity progression incorporates the external manifestation of coming out, but within a context of internal processes.

The sociological analogue to identity in the coming-out process is the concept "homosexual role." Identifying the self as homosexual refers not so much to the psychologist's notion of identity as an internal condition but to the individual's acceptance of membership in a socially proscribed and defined class labeled "homosexual" (McIntosh, 1968).[1] An individual could thus act in a homosexual fashion but not identify himself or herself with the socially constructed phenomenon of homosexuality. Similarly, Dank (1971) noted the significance of coming out within a social context, but his definition distinguished identifying oneself as homosexual—necessitating a new cognitive category of sexual identity and self-

---

[1]Whitam (1977) refuted the contention that homosexuality is a role: "While a role, as it is ordinarily understood, may be ascribed or achieved, children are neither socialized into the 'homosexual role' nor do they rationally choose it" (p. 1). Homosexuality, to Whitam, is a sexual orientation and thus neither a condition nor a role.

acceptance (although the two do not necessary occur together)—from the disclosure of that information to others. The public expression of coming out, according to Dank, signifies to the individual the end of the identity search. Thus, many sociologists separate the notions of acceptance of the homosexual role and the public expression of the homosexual role.

Identity Plus Disclosure

As best exemplified by the theoretical model of Cass (1979, 1984), the most usual solution to the discrepancies in definitions is to include both self-recognition and disclosure to others in the coming-out process. For example, Simon and Gagnon (1967) viewed coming out as the intersection of self-recognition of one's identity as a homosexual and the initial exploration of the homosexual community. De Monteflores and Schultz (1978) defined coming out as

> the developmental process through which gay people recognize their sexual preferences and choose to integrate this knowledge into their personal and social lives. A number of experiences are critical in this process: The awareness of same-sex attractions, first homosexual experience, coming out in the gay world, labeling oneself as gay or homosexual, coming out to friends, family, and co-workers, and coming out publicly. (p. 59)

Sophie (1985/1986) noted the difficulty in defining coming out, manifested not only among social scientists but also among gay males and lesbians:

> For some, it is intrapersonal and means the moment they realized that they were homosexual. For others, it denotes the time between the realization and an open or public acknowledgement of the fact. And for yet others, it is a composite of the two and includes the most painful moment: Disclosure to parents and family. (p. 31)

Harry and DeVall's (1978) solution was to split the two components, measuring "self-definition" as the age one first defined the self as gay or lesbian and "behavioral coming out" as the age one came out, without defining for their subjects what this meant. Each subject used his or her own terms. But it remains a rather unsatisfactory solution because it leaves many unanswered questions, including the nature of the relationship between identity and disclosure. In their study the correlation between the two was .65, indicating a significant amount of overlap but with some measurable distinction between the two. That is, the two did not occur during the same year for all individuals.

McDonald (1984) also found overlap but not perfect congruency between the two concepts. Those most out of the closet (those open in social situations and who did not pass as heterosexual) had the highest level of identity congruency—an integration of sexual behaviors, feelings, fantasies, and self-image—and were most "totally homosexual."

Others have combined the internal and external to divide research subjects into various categories. For example, four identity groups were distinguished on the basis of sexual attraction and behavior, patterns of socialization, chronological identity milestones, and identity disclosure (Cohen-Ross, 1985). Miller (1978) grouped his homosexual husbands into four classifications based on issues of self-recognition and public disclosure: trade (engages in homosexual behavior but no self-recognition as homosexual), homosexual (self-recognition but no public identity), gay (self-recognition with limited public knowledge), and faggot (self-recognition with public identity).

Issues involving the self are generally portrayed to be early processes, and once they have transpired then the individual is prepared to tell others. Although there is a certain intuitive feeling that this basic sequence is probably correct, there are exceptions: Those without self-recognition of their true sexual orientation who are known as gay or lesbian by others, those who are thrust out before they are psychologically ready (e.g., an early pubescent male caught sexually playing with a male cousin), and those who know that they are lesbian or gay but either never disclose to anyone except sexual partners or remain a virgin (e.g., a few nuns and priests). Weinberg (1978) noted, however, that most men are "doing" before "being," that is, engaging in homosexual behavior before defining the self as gay. Thus, many men disclose their homosexuality to another, the sexual partner, before the identity process has progressed very far.

Summary

A number of models have been proposed that combine coming out to self and to others. Examples include the following:

- Pre-coming out, coming out, exploration, first relationships, integration (Coleman, 1982);
- Sensitization, signification–disorientation/dissociation, coming out, commitment (Plummer, 1975; Troiden, 1979);
- Identity confusion, identity comparison, identity tolerance, identity acceptance, identity pride, identity synthesis (Cass, 1979);
- First conscious homosexual instinctive tendencies, repression and reemergence, homosexual contacts, self-perception as homosexual (Reiche & Dannecker, 1977).

These models form the basis for the discussion of the coming-out process in this chapter.

SENSITIZATION

Feeling Different

The origins of feeling somehow different from others are unclear. D'Emilio (1983, p. 20) noted that "initially their [gays and lesbians] sexuality created a profound, even disturbing, sense of difference from family, community, and society." Meager attempts may be made to name the attractions and feelings during the sensitization process. Relatively few adults, whether gay or straight, precisely recall when they first became aware of their sexual orientation. For many gay males and lesbians it seems more of a process of small realizations, filled with forward and backward steps, than an event or a sudden insight.

Whatever the path by which gay men and women arrived at a self-definition based on their sexuality, the labeling of one's sexual desires marked but the first step in a lifelong journey of discovery that offered challenges, perils, and rewards. "We stand in the middle of an uncharted, uninhabited country," Matthiessen wrote to his lover, Russell Cheney. (D'Emilio, 1983, p. 21)

With a sample of adults in the Netherlands (Sanders & De Koning, cited in Straver, 1976), two basic phases in homosexual identity development were delineated. The first, "feeling different," lasted a number of years but first reached consciousness during the first half of puberty between 12 and 15 years of age. At this time the realization that heterosexuality is the norm is continuously reinforced. Intra-psychic tensions increase when youths doubt their ability to meet the heterosexual obligations. Although some may be aware of their homosexual erotic attractions, others "only know that they are uninterested in intimate relationships with members of the opposite sex in their own age group, although they cannot indicate exactly what it is that they *do* want" (G. Sanders, 1980, p. 282). This feeling of being in a "vacuum" may have profound repercussions for issues of self-acceptance or self-rejection that evolve during later adolescence.

There is often an interlude between "first awareness" and the realization that this "feeling different" is homosexuality (Straver & Moerings, in Straver, 1976). Labeling these feelings may be accompanied by fears and anxieties of rejection and social isolation. A year or more usually elapses before this labeling is discussed with anyone else, usually first with a same-age friend.

However, many gay men and lesbians report feeling different at a very early age, long before puberty. The novelist Edmund White (1982) wrote, autobiographically, in *A Boy's Own Story,*

> *I see now that what I wanted was to be loved by men and to love them back but not to be a homosexual. For I was possessed with a yearning for the company of men, for their look, touch and smell, and nothing transfixed me more than the sight of a man shaving and dressing, sumptuous rites. It was men, not women, who struck me as foreign and desirable and I disguised myself as a child or a man or whatever was necessary in order to enter their hushed, hieratic company, my disguise so perfect I never stopped to question my identity. (p. 169)*

In Remafedi's (1987a) sample of gay youths, nearly one-third recalled an attraction to men that began from first memories in early childhood. For the rest, first awareness began in early to middle adolescence, ages 11 to 16 years.

Primarily as the result of Money and Ehrhardt's (1972) book on gender issues, it is generally accepted that sexual object choice as an integral component of gender identity is formed or predisposed at an early age, before 3 years. Consequently, sexual orientation may be present in some rudimentary form before the ability to reflect and label sexual feelings and attractions emerges. The vague, impressionistic sense of being different and isolated from peers, noted by Martin (1982), is characteristic of many preadolescent gay males and lesbians. In retrospect, without knowing why, they feel that somehow the difference is important (MacDonald, 1983; Robertson, 1981). These feelings and the accompanying process of self-searching are characteristic of the early stages of many theoretical coming-out models.

Troiden (1979) quoted a gay student who noted this sense of apartness during preadolescence: "I never felt as if I fit in. I don't know why for sure. I felt different. I thought it was because I was more sensitive" (p. 363). In his male sample, 72% felt this sense of being different. In an adult population (Bell, Weinberg, & Hammersmith, 1981a), considerably more gay males and lesbians than heterosexuals reported that they felt sexually different while growing up: 84% of the adult men and 74% of the adult women, but 11% and 10% of non-gay males and females, respectively. Reasons given for feeling different included lack of interest in members of the other sex, a desire to engage in activities or sports usually not attributed to one's sex, and possessing either feminine (for males) or masculine (for females) traits.

Source: Gender Nonconformity

The source of feeling different that has received the bulk of research attention is gender nonconformity (gender-atypical or cross-gendered behavior) in behaviors and interests. Green (1987) intensified this concern, focusing attention on boyhood cross-gendered behavior as clearly a correlate and perhaps a precursor to homosexuality. His theoretical "solution" was to suggest a developmental synthesis model that incorporated aspects of all classical explanations (physiological, psychoanalytic, and socialization) to account for the possible relation between boyhood femininity and adulthood homosexuality (see Chapter 10 in Green, 1987).

Regardless of the causative connection, the prevalence of childhood and adolescent gender-atypical behavior among gay and lesbian youth has been supported by a number of investigators. Early research (e.g., Bakwin, 1968; Green, 1974; Zuger, 1978) documented the coexistence of the two. Later, Bell et al. (1981a) posited gender nonconformity as a causative agent in the development of adult homosexuality, including

> homosexual activities and homosexual arousal before age 19, a sense of an explicitly sexual or at least gender-related difference from other boys [girls], and a delay in feelings of sexual attraction to girls [boys], as well as an adult homosexual preference. (p. 81)

Saghir and Robins (1973) simply noted the existence of gender nonconformity and its effects on the child and adolescent:

> Among boys destined to become adult male homosexuals, the prevalence of polysymptomatic effeminacy is very high. About two-thirds of the male homosexuals (67%), but only 3% of the male heterosexuals, described themselves as having been girl-like during childhood.
> Of the male homosexuals who fulfilled the criteria for polysymptomatic effeminacy in childhood, a large majority of them (77%) reported having had no male buddies, having avoided boys' games and having played predominantly with girls. All of them were called sissy and were teased about it by their schoolmates. It was an unhappy experience that most of them recalled very vividly. (pp. 18–19)

A "tomboyish" syndrome was four times more likely to be reported by homosexual than heterosexual girls (70% vs. 16%). The former tended to display an earlier onset of tomboy feelings and behaviors, show an aversion to dolls, and persist in masculine activities into adolescence and adulthood (Saghir & Robins, 1973).

At a very early age, either on a conscious or preconscious level, family members recognize that the gender-nonconforming child is different and that the atypicality may have implications for the child's sexual orientation (Coleman, 1982; Fling & Manosevitz, 1972). Conflicts within the family may escalate and the child, and then the adolescent, is faced with a number of decisions. Should he play it safe and pass as heterosexual, aware of his own deception and of living a lie?

Should she compartmentalize her life, separating her sexual self from all other activities and relationships? Should she disclose to others and risk the potential for ostracism, denial, and violence? The next step is frequently the most difficult.

SELF-RECOGNITION

Difficulties Encountered

Psychological and sociological models of the coming-out process frequently trace the development of these early feelings of alienation and uneasiness to full-scale inner and outer turmoil during adolescence. The growing realization that being different may mean being homosexual usually appears initially at the onset of puberty and then increases exponentially, especially from 10 to 18 years of age (Coleman, 1982; Jay & Young, 1979; Koodin et al., 1979; Remafedi, 1987a; Riddle & Morin, 1978; Robertson, 1981; Troiden, 1979). With a sample of 251 self-identified Utah gay men, Rodriguez (1988) reported that the group mean for awareness of same-sex attractions was in very early adolescence (11.1 years). Same-sex erotic fantasies occurred at 13.9 years, and labeling of feelings as homosexual was delayed until 16.2 years. First consensual homosexual orgasm followed soon thereafter (16.9 years), but labeling self as homosexual (20.6 years) and as gay (22.9 years) were much later events. The largest percentage of male adults, 41%, in Spada's (1979) study recalled that they first knew they were attracted to other males between 10 and 14 years; 20%, between 6 and 9 years; and 15%, between 15 and 18 years. On the other hand, other data (G. Sanders, 1980) suggest that this initial recollection occurred predominantly during the second half of puberty. Relatively few, less than 20%, of 789 West German gay male adults recognized feeling homosexual before 13 years of age (Reiche & Dannecker, 1977). The percentages increased sharply until 18 years and then leveled until 99% recognition at age 30 years. These feelings have "nothing in common with certainty, whatever form this certainty may take, or even with acceptance of one's own homosexuality" (p. 44). Not until 3 years later, at a mean age of 19.4 years, were the gay men essentially willing to perceive themselves as homosexuals. The mean age of self-identification in a group of 29 male youths was 14 years (Remafedi, 1987a).

The inconsistencies among the reports may be due to variations in the question asked (first feelings of attraction, labeling the feelings as homosexual, self-acknowledgment, etc.), cohort, characteristics of the sample (e.g., religion, rural–urban, social class, etc.), and perhaps other variables. Better methodologies and documentation are needed on this point. Regardless, the repercussions of this sexual awareness are usually considered to be fairly severe. Many gay and lesbian adults recall that as adolescents they were social isolates, loners, and outcasts. Compared to heterosexuals, they ranked low on social involvement, number of friends, popularity, dating, and participation in same-sex games (Bell et al., 1981a, 1981b; Grellert, 1982).

A number of authors have described defenses that adolescents develop to protect themselves. Tripp (1975) suggested in *The Homosexual Matrix* that gay males frequently use three systems of denial: assume the masculine role in homosexual sex; claim innocence because of drunkenness, drugs, sleep, etc.; and excuse it as no more than a "special friendship." The strategies adopted by adolescents to cope with these sexual feelings may vary considerably:

1. Rationalization (Cass, 1979; Plummer, 1981; Troiden, 1979): "Something I'll outgrow," "I did it because I was lonely," "Just a means to earn money," or "I was drunk/high."
2. Relegation to insignificance (Cass, 1979; Reiche & Dannecker, 1977; Troiden, 1979): "It is just sexual experimentation or curiosity that is natural at my age" or "Did it only as a favor for a friend."
3. Compartmentalization of sexual desire (de Monteflores & Schultz, 1978; Malyon, 1981; Martin, 1982): "I mess around with other boys/girls but that does not make me a faggot/dyke" or "I just love her and not all women."
4. Withdrawal from provocative situations to remain celibate or asexual (Cass, 1979; Lee, 1977; G. Sanders, 1980): "I'm saving myself for the right girl/boy."
5. Denial, frequently engaging in heterosexual dating or sexual behavior (Bell et al., 1981a; Cass, 1979; Martin, 1982; Reiche & Dannecker, 1977; G. Sanders, 1980): "I can't be gay, I've had a girlfriend/boyfriend for years and I like her/ him."
6. Redirection of energies to other efforts, such as intellectual or work pursuits (G. Sanders, 1980).

Malyon (1981), a clinical psychologist, outlined three adaptation modes that are the most frequent responses to the dilemma of being a homosexual adolescent (from least to most satisfactory adaptation). The first is repression of same-sex desires. Eventually, of course, the impulses must emerge, which may elicit panic or cause a major disruption of established coping strategies. The youth has had little opportunity to integrate homosexual desires with his or her identity. The second adaptation mode, suppression of homosexual impulses, often results in a temporary developmental moratorium. Identity formation is truncated because the adolescent attempts to pass as heterosexual, possibly leading to underachievement in school, unhappy heterosexual relations, a chronic psychological disequilibrium, and a biphasic or secondary adolescence during the third or fourth decades of life when he or she finally comes out. The third option is disclosure to self and others. But there are many hurdles yet to overcome. Remaining in the heterosexual community frequently involves estrangement and confusion, while a move to the lesbian or gay communities may precipitate a separation from or conflict with parents. Such a step also requires a premature assumption of adult social roles and responsibilities (Malyon, 1981).

During this time it is frequently difficult to assist the adolescent because the gay youth cannot ask for or will not accept assistance with a problem that for him does not exist. The young lesbian cannot disclose her inner turmoil to others because the tasks at hand are so nebulous and so intensely personal that she experiences "identity confusion" or an "existential crisis" (Cass, 1979; de Monteflores & Schultz, 1978). This process of "slowly surrendering" to the deviant identity entails weighing the costs to one's psychic self and one's relations with others, especially with family and friends (Coleman, 1982; Lee, 1977; MacDonald, 1983).

G. Sanders (1980) and Straver (1976) noted various adolescent reactions to the realization that the label *homosexual* applies to the self. One response is, "I can't keep it at bay any longer," but the youth remains "inwardly disapproving, and there is little motivation to adapt his social behaviour to the now recognized preference" (Straver, 1976, p. 129). Others feel a sense of liberation but are faced with societal stigma. Three forms of behavior may intervene before full acceptance is achieved:

1. A return to previous behavior, resisting the "deviant inclinations" and rejecting emerging homosexual feelings and desires;
2. A double life, which entails presenting an external socially acceptable form of behavior while inwardly being reconciled to homosexual feelings and becoming secretively immersed in aspects of a gay/lesbian life-style (Colgan, 1987; Straver, 1976); and
3. An attempt at social integration with the immediate environment that includes the "deviant pattern."

The double life option is most likely to result in low self-acceptance, inward turmoil, overseparation, and low levels of intimacy with others (Colgan, 1987).

Gender Differences in Coming Out

The vast majority of the coming-out models and empirical investigations are based on gay males and not lesbians. de Monteflores and Schultz (1978) suggested several ways in which the sexes differ:

1. Gay males sexually act on their homosexual feelings earlier after they become aware of same-sex attractions.
2. Homosexual behavior usually occurs for lesbians after an intellectual understanding of the term "homosexual"; gay males, before such an understanding.
3. Lesbians avoid self-identifying as homosexual by emphasizing their feelings ("My relationship with her is special and unique to only her"); gay males, as indicated earlier, avoid such self-identification by denying their feelings.
4. A self-label as homosexual is more threatening to males.
5. Coming out is more likely to be a political decision among lesbians.

Apparently, lesbians come out at a slightly older age than gay males, perhaps because of the extended time necessary for them to connect the "feeling different" with same-sex erotic feelings and behaviors. There is cross-cultural support for this gender difference. In the Netherlands (G. Sanders, 1980) boys became aware of their same-sex attraction feelings (median age = 13 years) and their homosexuality (median age = 15 years) earlier than girls (median ages = 16 and 18 years, respectively). Some (Bell et al., 1981a; Kinsey, Pomeroy, Martin, & Gebhard, 1953) suggested that in actuality there are fewer lesbians to come out; on the other hand, bisexuality may be more of an option for women than it is for men, thus reducing the number of lesbians in the population or prolonging the coming-out process ("I know I am attracted to men so I can't be a lesbian").

Another explanation is that because it is easier for females than males to pass as straight (Gagnon & Simon, 1973), there is less need for women to come out as lesbian. For example, Western culture allows women to display masculine behavior and to live together for an extended period of time without suspicion (Ponse, 1980). It is also not unusual for females to be portrayed as asexual: Two women expressing themselves physically or emotionally is more frequently labeled feminine than sexual behavior.

DISCLOSURE TO OTHERS

Roadblocks to Self-Labeling

Guilt feelings may cause an adolescent to delay defining himself or herself as homosexual for many years, perhaps waiting until after becoming a part of the lesbian/gay subculture (Harry & DeVall, 1978). Initially, a self-hating identity may be adopted, with an accompanying sexual moratorium (an inhibition of sexuality) (Cass, 1979). The lesbian adolescent may feel that she does not belong to society or to herself, or the gay male may take the self-pitying position, "Why me?!" The adolescent's task is a formidable one: recognizing that frequently articulated guidelines for future behavior, ideals, and expectations, meant to ensure a heterosexual identity, are not available or relevant to his or her life (Robertson, 1981). Furthermore, this loss is not replaced by a readily adopted and positive homosexual life. The continuity that an individual may have once had, based on a heterosexual model, between past and future may be forever gone, and the individual must now attempt to find new meanings and identities (Cass, 1979).

Because additional time may be necessary to integrate homosexuality with a sense of self, the youth may avoid threatening or provocative situations, keep tight control over any mannerisms and dress that might reveal her or his "true nature," and cultivate a deliberate heterosexual role (heterosexually dating). Rigg (1982, p. 827) noted, "Refuge may be taken in humor, both telling and laughing at anti-homosexual jokes, or in teasing others suspected of similar tendencies, to point the finger of suspicion in another direction." In such cases, Cass (1979) maintained, identity foreclosure is manifested, but the underlying psychological difficulties remain, to emerge later.

Passing as heterosexual is probably the most common adolescent adjustment to the fear of disclosure and its attendant feelings of guilt and anxiety (Dank, 1971; Lee 1977; Martin, 1982). Passing may lead to feelings of depression, awkwardness, and shame in interpersonal relations. Several humanistic clinical psychologists (Jourard, 1971; Maslow, 1954) have proposed that healthy personality development requires significant and substantial self-disclosure to others. A person establishes contact with the real self when the public self is made congruent with it (Jourard, 1971). Personal authenticity brings self-validation as a person of self-worth. To forego this, as in passing, engenders feelings of hypocrisy and self-alienation (Lee, 1977; Martin, 1982).

Not to pass, however, Coleman (1982) noted, can also be risky if one decides to disclose to others:

> If negative, it can confirm all the old negative impressions and can put a seal on a previous low self-concept. If positive, the reaction can start to counteract some of the old perceived negative feelings, permitting individuals to begin to accept their sexual feelings and increase their self-esteem. The existential crisis begins to resolve in a positive direction. (p. 34)

There are both personal and social repercussions:

> *It can propel a person whose homosexuality is of little salience for him into a homosexual*
> *role. Being publicly identified as homosexual means that others may relate to him in terms of*
> *this status rather than his other statuses and attributes. (Weinberg & Williams, 1974, p. 23)*

Although the process of coming out is difficult, the end result is usually positive, leading to identity synthesis and integration (Cass, 1979; Coleman, 1982); healthy psychological adjustment (Hammersmith & Weinberg, 1973); fewer feelings of guilt, loneliness, and need for psychiatric consultation (Dank, 1973); a deeper commitment to homosexuality through fusing gay sexuality and emotionality in a love relationship (Warren, 1974) or by viewing homosexuality as a preferred way of life (Troiden, 1979); integration through refining and maintaining both separation and attachment (Colgan, 1987); and a positive gay identity (McDonald, 1982).

THEORETICAL, EMPIRICAL, AND CLINICAL ISSUES

The inevitability of coming out as a necessary prerequisite to develop a self-conception of oneself as gay or lesbian is also challenged by two populations of gay men and lesbians. First, some report no memory of a coming-out process. They always knew, and because they were never "in the closet," there was never any need to come out, certainly not to the self and usually not to others. Others report that they have never experienced particular processes, such as the sudden revelation of one's homosexuality, that are purported to characterize the coming-out process. Weinberg (1984) criticized coming-out models on a number of points (e.g., understatement of the dynamic quality of coming out), but Coleman (1987, p. 18) asserted that they "serve as heuristic devices to understand better the developmental processes of identity development that do occur in some fashion."

Other unresolved issues include the linearity of the process within an individual's life. Is it not possible to backslide or to invert stages? There are also individual differences in the timing of the process, including absolute time in terms of age at reaching various set points and relative time in terms of reaching the points at ages earlier or later than previous generations of gay men and lesbians. Empirically, it appears that coming out is occurring earlier with each new cohort of gay men and lesbians, especially in urban, media-saturated, and collegiate communities. Research is needed that addresses whether coming out has recently become more compact, lasting a shorter period of time from start to finish. For example, I believe that it is no longer extremely rare for the coming-out process to begin shortly after pubertal onset and to be essentially completed (out to friends, family, and the public) by the end of adolescence. This can be attributable in large part to the recent visibility of lesbian and gay issues in society. The "unspeakable love" has appeared on television and in the movies, on the athletic fields and in the legislatures, on the bookshelves and in the medical literature, and, now, in teen-oriented magazines (July 1988 issue of *Sassy*).

There can be little dispute, however, as to the significance of coming-out milestones for some individuals. Many remember, and even celebrate, the anniversary of their coming out. Reiche and Dannecker (1977) noted,

> *The fact that they are actually able to remember the first consciously registered occurrence of the instinctual tendency is to be attributed only to the great effort expected from homosexuals due to their negative prominence in society. They feel compelled to account for an aspect of their biography, which is normally omitted in biographical reflections, even in the most honest ones. Nobody would seriously consider asking heterosexuals, when and why they became heterosexual. Homosexuals, on the other hand, ask themselves, at which point they became homosexual as often as they are asked about it. (p. 44)*

Books devoted primarily to revelatory stories (Heron, 1983; Stanley & Wolfe, 1980) document the pain, indecision, and occasionally violence, isolation, and alienation that accompany the coming-out process. For many others, however, the process is not particularly noteworthy or painful, certainly not the kind of revelation that will sell coming-out books.

In an article for the Chicago *Windy City Times,* Mel Wilson (1987) wrote of the the significance of coming out:

> *There is no agreement on the exact meaning of the words "coming out" but in all our conversations we seem able to put dates on the "event." By some sort of tacit consensus we never challenge the meaning of the term. "Coming out" is the common, shared bonding experience of gay men and lesbians, and yet for each of us it is a totally unique and singular experience . . . an experience that, once begun, never ends.*
>
> *It is because "coming out" is not easy that it forms a central marker in our lives: a dividing line of the "before" and "after." Gay men and lesbians "come out" for a lot of reasons—by force, for political objectives, for pride [or spite]—but there is only one "good" way to "come out" and that is to come out for ourselves. When we do, our lives become irretrievably altered— so altered, in fact, that we can't stop telling everyone we can find about it . . . over and over to the point that they either "come out" themselves, if they want to, or get as far away from us as possible if they don't. . . .*
>
> *For every individual, "coming out" is a singular experience: a choice between the lady and the tiger, a choice to abandon deception and deceit, a watershed in life. "Coming out" is a choice that is personal, sometimes public, and always political. It is not a point in time, but is instead a continuum. It is a beginning to making the world whole. It is the first step in claiming our place. (p. 8)*

Troiden (1989) cataloged various "facilitating factors" that ease the transition to a homosexual identity: education, supportive friends and family, young age, no heterosexual but some homosexual sexual experiences, and gender atypicality. Few if any of these have been systematically investigated.

The psychologically and sociologically best time to come out to oneself and to others is an issue few have addressed. Apparently, coming out to oneself at a relatively early age but revealing that identity only to select others until the environment is positive and supportive (usually after high school) is best. Such individuals avoid the negative repercussions of being known as gay or lesbian in the junior and senior high school settings without facing the negative psychological consequences of denial, repression, suppression, rationalization, etc. They take their time, disclosing their sexual identity to "safe" persons who give necessary social and psychological support. In the process they learn crisis competence and develop an internal sense of self-respect and ego integrity that prepares them to face the cruelty of a homophobic peer society (Coleman, 1982; Kimmel, 1978; Malyon, 1981).

Thus, there is clearly a need for supportive services for the gay or lesbian individual and for those who, when confronted with the news, perceive that they are adversely affected, such as parents. There is a growing "coming out right" advice literature for youths and their loved ones (noted in Chapter 8). There are also support groups for gay and lesbian youth (e.g., the Hetrick-Martin Institute in New York City, Horizons in Chicago, and the Minnesota Task Force on Gay and Lesbian Youth in Minneapolis) and for their friends and parents (e.g., National Federation of Parents and Friends of Lesbians and Gays).

It is important to detail the coming-out process, even if one denies its universality, because of its importance in understanding and appreciating the conditions faced by gay and lesbian youth growing up in today's environment. Many have recited the day-to-day pains and crises that lesbian and gay adolescents frequently encounter with others, both those loved and those not. Our ignorance of these issues of coming out has had and will continue to have consequences for our youth. As noted by Harry and DeVall (1978, p. 79), "For many . . . the conflicts and confusions experienced in the teen-age closet take several years, perhaps a lifetime to overcome." They may feel different and alienated, fail to integrate and develop a sense of identity in a hostile environment, constantly fear exposure of the innermost secret, and face peer ridicule if they are "inappropriately" effeminate/masculine.

The theoretical, empirical, and clinical issues raised in this chapter highlight many of the coming out concerns of youth and researchers alike. In Chapter 7, several of these issues are explored in more depth, forming the basis for the research questions focused on coming out that are reported in this book.

4

Research Design and Procedures

OVERVIEW

As is true with any research project, difficult decisions were made in regard to the population of youth sampled, research procedures, and measures given to the youths. One research project cannot provide sufficient data to answer the many research needs that were noted in the literature reviewed in the previous chapters. There were, however, particular research priorities that I accepted. In designing a research project to address issues of self-esteem and coming out among gay and lesbian youth there were a number of seemingly insurmountable obstacles. The final resolution, described in this chapter, is far from ideal. It represents a compromise of the model study that I intended to undertake and the realities that I faced once the research design and procedures were actually implemented. These will be briefly recounted, along with particular research priorities that guided this study.

PROBLEMS AND PRIORITIES

The primary research goal was to assess the psychological well-being of a diversified population of gay and lesbian youth, especially those seldom involved in research on homosexuality. I wanted neither a New York City nor a San Francisco sample, both of which are well represented in previous research, but one that drew gay males and lesbians from other sectors of our society. It was important, because of my interest in issues of self-esteem, to include a wide spectrum of the gay and lesbian youth population, especially in terms of the coming-out process and sexual orientation. It is too rare in research on homosexuality to include "closet" cases and those who maintain some heterosexual interest. Other aspects of diversity among youth—religion, race, social class, educational level, family situation, sexual experience, political ideology, and love affairs—were also considered important issues to examine.

A second priority was to explore self-esteem and self-disclosure during the years of the life course when issues of identity are central for healthy development. Although self-evaluation is a developmental issue from the first notion of self in infancy and one that lasts throughout the life course, the vast majority of psychological and sociological research has focused on the teen and late adolescent years because of the commonly held assumption that it is during this time when reflections on the self are most intense. It is also the time when many individuals begin the process of reconciling erotic attractions and sexual identity. I wanted to understand feelings of self-worth and the coming-out process among adolescents and youths who define themselves to some degree as homosexual.

This raised a difficult issue: what it means to be homosexual. A necessary first consideration in any research on homosexuality must include conceptual and operational definitions of sexual orientation (Coleman, 1987; Shively, Jones, & De-Cecco, 1983/1984). Because my intent was to explore developmental issues from a psychological and not a biological or sociocultural perspective, I chose "self-identification" as my conceptual definition. That is, if a respondent defined himself or herself on the Kinsey Heterosexual-Homosexual Rating Scale (Kinsey et al., 1948) (the operational instrument used) as being at least "significantly homosexual" (Kinsey's 2–6) then he or she was included as a study participant. Respondents were not asked what "significantly homosexual" meant to them—for example, sexual activity, erotic attraction, affectionate attachments, or cultural labels (Shively et al., 1983/1984). This should be viewed as a limitation of the present study because there is great diversity in regard to the meaning of homosexuality. Researchers have few clues as to the significance of these meanings for their dependent variables. Relationships among variables reported in this book might depend to some degree on this conceptual breadth of designating study participants. Because the present research was construed as a broad-based, descriptive project, this inclusive definition seemed justified. Future studies asking more in-depth questions of lesbian and gay youth might do well to specify the meaning that "being homosexual" has for the individual (Coleman, 1987). In addition, this would imply use of a more finely tuned instrument than the Kinsey scale.

Although there is an almost endless list of variables one could use to describe a gay or lesbian population or to predict level of self-esteem and coming out, those included in this study were of interest because past theoretical speculations or empirical research indicated that they were appropriate variables to investigate. It was also important to use a research instrument that was relatively simple and brief to insure the cooperation of research participants, especially if young adolescents and a diversified sample were to be included.

Finally, it was necessary to assume a research position between that of a sociological survey and a clinical psychologist, probably reaching neither the former's breadth nor the latter's depth. A large-scale survey method was ruled out because of my prior decision to include those who were not yet public in their declaration of sexual orientation, who were not "urban gays," and who were not readily accessible except by special effort. The difficulty in finding large numbers of lesbian and gay youths appeared formidable. On the other hand, I did not want to adopt a clinical research strategy of case studies that would severely limit any generalizations to a wider population. Because of the potential sensitivity of the research issues, a questionnaire that could be completed and submitted anonymously increased the possibility of privacy and honesty in responding. Self-report procedures are not my favorite research strategy because they assume that respondents are able and willing to tell the truth (see Savin-Williams, 1987a), but other research strategies such as observation of naturalistic behavior, interviews, and ratings would not (a) answer the initial fundamental research questions that I wanted to address, (b) provide bountiful baseline data that are necessary for giving direction to future research on gay and lesbian youth, or (c) be feasible from a practical point of view.

My goal was to survey youths after the onset of puberty and before the attainment of adult status, which was set at 23 years to allow for some age spread and to include those who were in or had just finished college. Data collection began on July 1, 1983, and concluded 5 months later on December 1, 1983, with 255 questionnaires completed. To increase sample size and diversity, 62 additional questionnaires were later collected from participants of a regional gay and lesbian student conference in Ithaca, New York.

The research project was reviewed by the Cornell University Human Subjects Committee. Their concerns were twofold: (a) maintaining the confidentiality of the respondents, which was insured with the procedures described below; and (b) preventing heterosexual youths from being accidentally subjected to the questionnaire. This latter concern I could not guarantee but would try to minimize.[1]

MEASURES

Gay and Lesbian Questionnaire

In reaching a decision on an appropriate questionnaire to distribute to youth, I was influenced by Bell's (1975) plea that researchers create "not yet another" gay questionnaire. In examining the available options I was struck with the realization that there were few if any designed for adolescent aged gay males and lesbians. My solution was to borrow from previously used questionnaires. The Blumstein–Schwartz (1983) Couples Survey Questionnaire incorporated many of the issues that were of interest to me, and they were kind enough to grant permission to modify their questionnaire for my purposes. Additional items were included from a questionnaire developed by Weinberg and Williams (1974). Finally, several adolescent-oriented questions were added concerning parenting, love affairs, physical development, and athletics. Completing the Gay and Lesbian Questionnaire (GAL Q) took 15 to 30 minutes.

Reliability data have not been provided by the authors of these two questionnaires. Because all participants in the current study were guaranteed anonymity, reliability data could not be collected from the youths included in this research. However, the semester after data collection was completed I asked my undergraduate class on theory and research on homosexuality to take the GAL Q. One month later they completed the GAL Q a second time, with the explanation that I wanted the class to discuss the questionnaire. Through use of the sociodemographic information provided on the first page—primarily sex, age, religion, and town reared in—I was able to match the two questionnaires of 10 gay males and 9 lesbians in the class. I excluded questionnaires from straight students in the class. These 19 served as the reliability data reported in this book.

Because all potential variables that might be related to self-esteem and coming out could not be examined, choices needed to be made in constructing the GAL Q. Variables were included if, on the basis of psychological or sociological theory, previous research with gay or lesbian populations had indicated that they were related to either self-esteem or coming out and if they were of particular interest

---

[1]In a letter to the Committee I objected to what appeared to me to be subtle homophobia: "Gay people are continually being bombarded with a heterosexual world, and few consider our rights or sensitivities. The Committee seems deeply concerned with protecting "straight" people from exposure to my gay-oriented questionnaire. They might be offended or hurt, or feel "put down" because the distributor of the GAL Q thought they were gay. God forbid! Yet, where is the Committee's protection of gay people from exposure to heterosexually oriented questionnaires, interviews, and surveys? Might gays be offended by the assumption of the distributor that they are straight? Most instruments/measures you approve have a biased heterosexual orientation. Did you become equally concerned with those as you did the GAL Q?"

because of their relevance for self-development during the years of adolescence and youth. This evidence is reviewed in the next chapter.

Unfortunately, because of space limitations on the questionnaire and the priority that was placed on casting a wide net of variables that are important for issues of self-esteem and coming out, in most cases only one question assessed a construct. As any methodologist well knows, this is far from the ideal state. Thus, this limitation must be considered when reading the research findings reported in this book.

Variables included in the GAL Q assessed one of seven major clusters that were considered by theory or past research to differentiate self-esteem and coming-out level. For example, age, education, education-age class, community, occupational status, and onset of puberty form the items in the sociodemographics cluster. Other clusters were attitudes and interests, gay-related activities, perceived support from family and friends, love affairs, self-descriptions, and sense of self-worth.

Rosenberg Self-Esteem Scale

One of the most frequently used measures of adolescent self-esteem is the Rosenberg Self-Esteem Scale (RSE; Rosenberg, 1979). The RSE is a 10-item scale that addresses issues of global self-esteem (e.g., "On the whole, I am satisfied with myself"), explicitly distinct from specific contexts such as time of day or recent events or activities. On a 4-point scale, from *strongly agree* to *strongly disagree*, respondents indicate the degree to which the five positively stated and five negatively stated sentences characterize them. The scoring method is a four-step system that has a structural reliability of .89, far superior to procedures developed by Rosenberg and modified by Simmons (Rosenberg, 1979; Simmons & Blyth, 1987). Interitem reliability and the RSE's correlation with other self-report self-esteem scales are consistently high (Demo, 1985; Savin-Williams & Demo, 1984). Test–retest reliability with the sample of 19 was quite high at .88. Several distinct advantages of the RSE contribute to its ideal use with adolescents: the simply worded and easily understood statements, an average completion time of 2 to 5 minutes, comparability of results with many other populations of adolescents, and its suitability with a wide age range (from age 11 years through adulthood).

Coming Out

Assessing the degree to which one has come out to others is problematic because there are few standardized and validated instruments. As noted in Chapter 3, existing measures are plentiful in number but also diverse in the construct that they assess. Early investigations relied solely on criteria based on sexual behavior for discriminating between overt and covert gay males and lesbians. Later studies operationalized overtness according to one's willingness to disclose sexual orientation to a variety of others, such as employers, friends, acquaintances, and family members. Ferguson and Finkler (1978) suggested that both being known about by others and a willingness to disclose one's sexual identity are important measures of overtness. Thus, they combined the two for a composite measure of overtness that included both attitudinal and behavioral aspects of overtness. Overtness was operationalized by asking respondents to rate 37 items in terms of (a) the degree of comfort they felt with the suggested behavior and (b) their actual behavior. Among the behaviors listed were disclosing one's sexual identity to an employer, telling one's parents about a same-sex affair, and performing oral sex with a member of the same sex.

In this study two variables measured coming out. The first, the attitudinal dimension, assessed the extent to which the youths were willing to disclose their sexual orientation to others. On the basis of the Weinberg-Williams (1974) questionnaire, an item on the GAL Q asked respondents how much they care whether heterosexuals know they are gay: 4 = "I do not care who knows I am gay," 3 = "There are a few heterosexuals I do not want to know I am gay," 2 = "There is a large number of heterosexuals I do not want to know I am gay," and 1 = "I do not want any heterosexuals to know I am gay." A score of 4 represents those most overt, most willing to disclose their sexual preference to all, and a score of 1 represents those most covert or least willing to disclose.

The second, behavioral variable, knownness to select others, was constructed from a question asking the youths whether their mother, father, closest sibling, best heterosexual male and female friend, and academic advisor know that they are lesbian/gay. For each, the youths answered with one of the following responses: 4 = "Definitely knows and we have talked about it," 3 = "Definitely knows but we have never talked about it," 2 = "Probably knows or suspects," 1 = "Does not know or suspect."

The overtness assessments were quite stable in the reliability group over the course of a month. All 19 subjects gave identical ratings for being out to father, sibling, and best female friend on the two self-reports. At Time 2 one male was less out and one female more out to their mothers, one female was less out to her professor, and one male was less out and one female more out to a best heterosexual male friend. The last individual apparently came out totally to her "boyfriend" during the month (from "does not know or suspect" to "we have talked about it"). One male and one female reported they were slightly more publicly out at Time 2. Thus, of 130 opportunities (19 subjects × 7 overtness measures − 3 missing data points), the reliability sample gave identical ratings on 123 (95%) occasions. Of the seven exceptions, four were progressions to greater disclosure.

It should be noted that these assessments are not objective measures of a youth's being known about; for example, a youth may think that the parents know about her or his homosexuality when in fact they do not, or vice versa. Thus, this measure taps only a subjective judgment of whether or not others know about one's sexual orientation.

GAY AND LESBIAN QUESTIONNAIRE

Table 4.1 summarizes where we recruited the sample of youths.

Community Picnic

The Common Ground is an Ithaca, New York, gay bar noted for its diversity in clientele, with patrons representing many sexual orientations, ethnicities, and ages and both sexes equally. Every summer the Common Ground sponsors a picnic, the proceeds of which are donated to the gay and lesbian community (AIDS Task

Table 4.1 Where the sample was recruited

Source	Males		Females		Total	
	n	%	*n*	%	*n*	%
A community picnic sponsored by the Common Ground bar	13	6	10	10	23	7
Campus gay meetings on university campuses	44	21	5	5	49	15
Female undergraduates who gave questionnaires to their friends and their networks	19	9	37	36	56	18
Male undergraduates who gave questionnaires to their friends and their networks	69	32	9	9	78	25
Contact persons in other states	27	13	16	16	43	14
Attendees of a North-East Conference of Gay and Lesbian Student Activists	42	20	20	19	62	20
Cornell University's sexuality class	0	0	6	6	6	2
Total	214		103		317	

Force, athletic teams, etc.). Gay men and lesbians who attend this community event come from the local community and colleges and from nearby towns and cities such as Binghamton, Corning, Elmira, Rochester, and Syracuse.

A box with blank GAL Qs and pencils was placed by the food table with a sign that advertised the research project. A box for completed questionnaires was on the other side. During, in between, and after such activities as eating, drinking, playing volleyball and softball, and watching the wet T-shirt and wet shorts contests, respondents completed the GAL Q.

More than 200 people were in attendance but because most who were present were over 23 years of age, relatively few of the GAL Qs were usable. It was not possible to compute a return rate at the picnic because I had no way of knowing how many of those under 23 years of age saw the sign, and of those who did, how many responded.

Campus Gay Meetings

At the three campus meetings, 100% sampling (all who were given a questionnaire completed it) was achieved. I described the research project at the University of Minnesota campus gay and lesbian meeting. All 15 males who were present under the age of 23 years responded positively; all females who were present were over 23 years of age. At a wine and cheese reception for returning and new gay and lesbian students in Binghamton, New York, each of the 13 males present was given a GAL Q. He either completed it during the evening or mailed it to me the next day. At Iowa State University a package of GAL Qs was sent to a contact person, a friend of one of the undergraduate research assistants. At a regular weekly meeting the 5 women and 16 men present completed the GAL Q.

Although these meetings were open to both men and women, they were strikingly male dominated. The major objective in distributing the GAL Qs to these quite divergent geographic locations was to enhance diversity in the population sampled. This was achieved in some part by this technique.

Friendship Networks

Almost one-half of the total number of questionnaires that we collected came from our friendship networks. We gave the GAL Qs to friends and asked those friends to distribute extra questionnaires to their friends. As might be expected, our networks tended to be same sex. Because of the low number of women that were responding in early returns, I made a special request of the female research assistants to recruit lesbians. Unfortunately, most lesbians they knew were over the age of 23 years. The GAL Qs were either returned immediately to one of us or, as was the case in nearly three-quarters of these occasions, returned in a preaddressed, sealed envelope.

I asked no further information of the research assistants concerning to whom they gave the GAL Qs, in order to maintain anonymity. My goal was not only diversity, assuming that our friendship networks varied, but also to include those who were not "out" to many others. This was the most anonymous technique and was preferred, it was our impression, by those most uncomfortable with public knowledge of their sexual orientation. Thus, the largest number of questionnaires were given directly to our acquaintances or to our friends' friends. Of the approximately 300 questionnaires we distributed, 134 were returned; four individuals refused directly, citing opposition to research on homosexuality. The rest were either not given by our friends to others, were discarded or lost, or were not completed or returned to us.

Mail-Away Sources

To increase geographic diversity—that is, to include non-upstate New York youths—the six of us sent 10 questionnaires to a friend in another state. The friends were requested to give the questionnaires to gay men and lesbians they knew who were 23 years or younger. We received positive responses from states in the Midwest (Missouri, Iowa), South (Mississippi), North Central (Wisconsin, Minnesota), and East (New England communities). Nearly one-fifth of our sample was derived from these mail-away sources. Of the 60 questionnaires we sent to our friends, 43 were returned completed; the others were returned blank because, we assumed, they were never distributed. Although our friends reported they had only several refusals, we had no independent means of verifying this.

Activist Conference

Ithaca, New York, was the setting for the second annual North-East Conference of Gay and Lesbian Student Activists. Of the 180 students registered, 67 attended a workshop that I conducted; during this time the GAL Qs were distributed. Sixty-two students returned a completed questionnaire. The students were from 27 colleges in New York, Massachusetts, Rhode Island, Pennsylvania, New Jersey, West Virginia, Connecticut, and Vermont.

Human Sexuality Class

Finally, a few questionnaires were returned from a human sexuality class taught at Cornell University by Dr. Andrea Parrot. GAL Qs were distributed to the class of 200, but only 6 female students rated themselves as a Kinsey 2–6. We have no knowledge of the percentage of youths in the class, gay male or lesbian, who failed to complete the questionnaire. We were surprised, however, at the relatively small number of usable GAL Qs that were received from this source, especially because the course has a positive reputation among lesbian and gay students on the Cornell campus.

Return Rate

Given these data collection techniques it is not possible to compute an exact or even an approximate return rate. Although the research topic should have evoked a poor response rate because homosexuality is frequently considered sociologically deviant and psychologically covert or unhealthy (Hedblom & Hartman, 1980), our participating population proved to be most cooperative. This was due, I believe, to the research strategy that emphasized a personal and confidential approach. Only rarely did someone object to the research; most were quite pleased to have fellow gay males and lesbians conduct the research.

STUDY PARTICIPANTS

Gay Males

Of the 317 respondents completing the questionnaire, 214 (68%) were gay males. They ranged in age from 14 to 23 years, with 74% between the ages of 19 and 22 years. See Table 4.2 for the distribution of ages.

Despite our attempts to solicit those not in college, many (75%) in the sample were college students during data collection; 15% had no college experience. Described in Table 4.3 is the educational status of the male sample when data were collected.

The male population was primarily Caucasian (90%) and diverse in religious affiliation: Catholic (34%), Protestant (33%), none (18%), Jewish (15%), and Eastern religions (1%). The ethnic minorities were Hispanic American (4%), African American (2%), Asian American (2%), Native American (1%), and international (1%).

When questioned concerning their hometown community, the gay males reflected a decidedly rural (21%) and small town (25%) flavor. The others were from medium-sized towns (26%), small cities (9%), and large metropolitan areas (19%). In terms of occupational status, the families of the gay males were classified as professional (37%), lesser professional/managerial (38%), or blue collar (18%).

Table 4.2 Distribution of ages of study participants

Age	n	% of total
	Gay males (n = 214)	
14–17	17	8
18	15	7
19	37	17
20	42	20
21	45	21
22	34	16
23	24	11
	Lesbians (n = 103)	
16–17	3	3
18	6	6
19	19	18
20	22	21
21	30	29
22	18	17
23	5	5

Table 4.3 Educational status of the sample

Category	Age	Years of education completed	n	% of total
	Gay males			
In school				
High school	14–17	8–11	9	4
College freshman	17–22	12	21	10
College sophomore/junior	17–23	13–14	75	35
College senior	20–23	15	47	22
Graduate student	21–23	16	18	8
Out of school				
No college	16–23	9–12	19	9
Some college	19–23	13–15	12	6
College graduate	21–23	16	13	6
	Lesbians			
In school				
High school	16	10	1	1
College freshman	17–19	12	5	5
College sophomore/junior	17–22	13–14	36	35
College senior	20–23	15	39	38
Graduate student	22–23	16	7	7
Out of school				
No college	19–22	12	6	6
Some college	19–21	13	5	5
College graduate	22–23	16	4	4

Lesbians

Lesbians comprised one-third ($n = 103$) of the sample. Most (85%) were between the ages of 19 and 22 years, with the youngest at 16 years and the oldest at 23 years representing the extreme points (See Table 4.2).

The vast majority (86%) of the lesbians were in college during data collection. The educational status of the lesbians is presented in Table 4.3.

Two Asian Americans, one Hispanic American, one African American, and one Native American were among the 103 lesbians in the study. More than 60% of the sample were Catholic (34%) or Protestant (31%). The rest were Jewish (17%), none (15%), or Eastern religions (3%).

The lesbians had a slightly less rural upbringing than the gay males. Although 12% grew up in rural areas, 59% were from either small- (29%) or medium- (30%) sized towns. Another 30% were raised in small cities (17%) or large metropolitan areas (13%). Most of the families of the lesbian sample were either professional (34%) or lesser professional/managerial (37%); there was, however, a large number (22%) of blue collar homes represented.

Reflection on the Participants

Although I was pleased with the number of youths who participated in the study, I was not satisfied with our recruitment of lesbians. They were far more difficult to find, despite our extra efforts. This shortage may reflect the lower number of lesbians in the population that has been reported by others (e.g., Bell, Weinberg, & Hammersmith, 1981a; Kinsey, Pomeroy, Martin, & Gebhard, 1953) or an indication that women come out at a later age.

The sample consisted of many highly educated late adolescents. Only 13% had no college experience and an additional 6% were college dropouts. This bias resulted from our techniques of data collection—for example, college campus meetings and our friendship networks. There were no local or nearby organizations that served the needs of noncollege teenagers that we could solicit for research participants. The recent research of Herdt, Boxer, and Irvin in Chicago (see Chapter 1) has filled this gap, at least with urban teenagers.

On the positive side, the sample included groups that have rarely appeared in previous studies of gay men and lesbians:

- adolescents under the age of 18 years (6%),
- youths with 12 or fewer years of education (11%),
- rural (18%) and small town (26%) lesbian and gay youth,
- Jews (15%),
- working-class lesbian and gay youth (18%),
- those who maintain significant heterosexual interest (22%),
- those not yet out to anyone (4%) or out to few others (27%).

In particular, I was pleased with the fairly sizable sample of rural/small town gay males and lesbians, especially given the dearth of research with this population that has been noted by D'Augelli and Hart (1987).

Chapter 5 reviews the previous empirical research conducted with populations of lesbians and gay males that investigated factors associated with self-esteem.

Research questions that emerged from this review were addressed in the current study. Chapter 6 includes a description of the present study's measures that assessed the relevant constructs, research findings from the present study that address these self-esteem issues, and a discussion and comparison of the present research results with previous research findings. The literature, present findings, and discussion of coming out are in Chapter 7. Chapter 8 is devoted exclusively to the role of the parents for the coming-out process and level of self-esteem. The final two chapters examine issues of gender differences, diversity, and the promise of being remembered and visible.

5

Predicting Self-Esteem

OVERVIEW

Because few investigators in the past have been concerned with lesbian and gay youth, by necessity one must turn to other evidence. Two sources are usually cited for empirical evidence of variables that are associated with or predict self-esteem: retrospective accounts of adults as they reflect on their adolescence and inferences from adult data. These strategies may not necessarily produce erroneous relationships if one accepts the view that self-esteem is essentially a stable characteristic of one's personality and thus not generally subject to high degrees of modification as the direct result of situational or environmental factors (Savin-Williams & Demo, 1984).

An important limitation was placed on the literature reviewed in this chapter: Only research in which the participants were gay men, lesbians, or bisexuals is considered. There is a large body of empirical studies that attempts to predict self-acceptance or self-esteem level on the basis of almost any conceivable variable. This literature is not summarized in this chapter for several reasons. First, I did not want to assume that self-esteem is related to the tested variables in the same manner that has been empirically demonstrated with heterosexual populations. Perhaps the developmental trajectory of evolving a sense of self-worth among lesbian and gay youth is in some way unique. Second, I wanted to avoid the danger of posing straight youth as a "control" or comparison group. To do so would imply that gay and lesbian youth were normal or psychologically healthy only when they were similar to or when they approached the relationships among variables characteristic of heterosexual youth. When they did not, then something must be wrong. Third, I was not willing to assume that I had sampled a "normal" or "random" subset of lesbian and gay youth. Therefore, it would be difficult to operationally define a comparable heterosexual sample. Thus, for both professional and political reasons, assumptions and implications of straight versus gay research were avoided.

SOCIODEMOGRAPHIC CHARACTERISTICS

Relatively few sociodemographic characteristics of the individual, such as age, education, pubertal onset, hometown community size, and parental occupational status have been systematically investigated as predictors of self-esteem among gay males and lesbians of any age. Yet, these class variables are important from an exploratory stance in that they may designate processes that are closely linked with self-esteem. The sparse literature on these topics provides a relatively weak basis for a formulation of testable hypotheses. Thus, research questions based on sociodemographic variables must be stated tentatively.

In regard to age, the vast majority of the research contrasts the self-esteem or self-satisfaction of middle-aged or elderly gay men and women with that of young adults. For example, a study by Weinberg and Williams (1974) contradicted the traditional stereotype of the elderly gay man as a lonely, depressed, and self-degrading individual. More than 1,000 New York City and San Francisco gay men participated in the study. There were no age-related differences in self-acceptance, and the older men (45 years or older) had somewhat higher well-being scores (stable self-concepts, worry less about exposure, little desire for psychiatric treatment) than other participants.

Harry and DeVall's Detroit study (1978) of 238 gay men, ranging in age from 18 to 50 years or older (20% older than 40 years), reported that age was unrelated to self-esteem. In his later Chicago sample of 1,556 gay men, Harry (1984) divided his sample into two groups: those currently or formerly in a relationship (89%) and those never in a relationship (11%). He found that in the latter group the percentage of men with low self-esteem rose from 54% among those under 25 years of age to 83% among those 45 years and older. For men who had or had had a relationship, there was a modest trend for self-esteem to increase with age.

Berger (1982) reported that with increasing age in his sample of gay males 40 years or older, self-acceptance and life satisfaction scores increased as well. He felt this was due to the greater likelihood that the senior gay male experienced good physical health, was integrated into the gay community, was less likely to conceal his homosexuality or to desire a change in his sexual orientation, and was involved in a relationship. Friend's (1980) sample of senior gay adults (M = 48 years) also reported a high degree of adjustment, as assessed by select self-esteem items. Ninety-one percent of the men said they had a number of good qualities, and 77% replied that they take a positive attitude toward the self.

Carlson and Steuer (1985) found no age effect on self-esteem in a correlation analysis with a sample of 165 gay men and 156 lesbians between the ages of 17 and 78 years. In fact, with age depression scores decreased among the homosexual men. In Cramer's (1986) sample of 93 gay males there was a positive, but nonsignificant, correlation between age and self-esteem level.

Although these studies are consistent in that they reveal either little or a slightly positive relationship between age and self-esteem, I have yet to discover an empirical study that examined self-esteem development as a function of age during the critical years of adolescence and youth. This is rather surprising given the general theoretical and empirical interest by developmentalists in adolescent self-esteem. Literally hundreds of articles have appeared in psychology and sociology journals examining this issue, encompassing many theoretical perspectives and assessment instruments—but always with an assumed heterosexual population. Thus, the gay and lesbian literature provides little guidance concerning the relationship between age and self-esteem among youth.

Similarly, the relationship between educational level and social class with self-esteem level has also been generally ignored. Harry and DeVall (1978) reported that the correlation between level of education attained, usually highly associated with occupational status, and self-esteem was quite low. In regard to social class Weinberg and Williams (1974) found, contrary to societal stereotypes, that upper social class gay men had higher levels of self-acceptance than middle and lower occupational status groups: "Thus, even if the homosexual in a high-status occupation faces greater strain associated with the way in which he manages his homosexuality, this would appear to be outweighed by the greater social psychological rewards associated with his social position" (Weinberg & Williams, 1974, p. 322). Similarly, lower class status lesbians were more anxious than higher status women (Ferguson & Finkler, 1978).

Size of hometown community was included because of concern, most recently expressed by D'Augelli and Hart (1987), with homosexism and lack of community support in nonurban settings. In rural areas, D'Augelli and Hart noted, there is seldom a visible gay support system, sufficient information about gay life, familial and friendship support of alternative life-styles, and opportunities to observe and acquire personal and social skills unique for lesbians and gay men. Thus, competence-building resources are limited in nonurban areas.

Pubertal onset, either in absolute or relative time, has been ignored in the homosexuality literature, aside from its potential causal role in the development of sexual orientation (e.g., Storms, 1981). Date of pubertal onset was included in this study because of its unique relevance for this age period in the life course.

Hypotheses

There is little evidence in the literature that sociodemographic factors contribute significantly to an increased understanding of self-esteem among gay and lesbian youth. It should be noted, however, that by and large these studies focused on an age group considerably older than those participating in the current study and on gay males and not lesbians. Nevertheless, it was proposed, on the basis of the literature reviewed above, that (a) age and pubertal onset would be unrelated to self-esteem; (b) those with high social status, with many years of education, and from urban areas would have more positive levels of self-esteem; and (c) in general, the sociodemographic variables would not be highly predictive of self-esteem.

ATTITUDES AND INTERESTS

Considering that the attitudes one has are frequently interrelated, several attitudes and interests were investigated in this study. Self-esteem is defined by many theorists, such as Rosenberg (1979) and Coopersmith (1967), as an attitude. Thus, it seems reasonable to assume that self-esteem is associated with other attitudes and interests that an individual has. For example, from a labeling perspective Weinberg (1983) proposed that an intricate association exists between the views an individual holds toward homosexuality and his or her self-evaluation level once the individual has identified with the label. Thus, "If an individual learns to view homosexuals negatively, guilt, fear, and ambivalence will accompany self-labeling as homosexual" (p. 36).

Deciding which attitudes to assess was based on two considerations. First, aside from religiosity, it was not possible to turn to the empirical literature for direction. An alternative, speculation derived from personal observations, was adopted. Gay men and lesbians most liberal, and thus most accepting of sexual minorities, in their sociopolitical outlook were perceived to be those most likely to also accept the self. This was explored by three questions: a general liberalism/conservatism continuum and specific questions in regard to support of the feminist movement and desire to have and raise children. Finally, a number of lesbian friends suggested that lesbians who play softball or basketball seem particularly self-assertive and self-assured. Thus I included questions on the Gay and Lesbian Questionnaire that assessed interest in and skill at sports.

One empirical study that examined religiosity in relation to self-esteem level found relatively few differences in self-acceptance levels between the more and less religious (Weinberg & Williams, 1974). On the basis of reports of gay men in three countries, including those living in New York City and San Francisco, Weinberg and Williams suggested that

> *among many homosexuals, some kind of accommodation between religious beliefs and sexual orientation is achieved. Some homosexuals may refuse to relate homosexuality to religious doctrine; they may simply not think about religion when involved in homosexual activities or vice versa. (p. 361)*

On the other hand, in a study of overt gay men and women (Clingman & Fowler, 1976), recruited primarily from the Gay Metropolitan Church (65%), gay bars, and friendship networks, church attendees had significantly higher levels of self-confidence than those who did not attend church. It is questionable, perhaps, that church attendance is an adequate proxy for religiosity, that is, that those who go to church are more religious than those who do not.

Hypotheses

Because I found no study that examined the influence on self-esteem of political ideology (liberal–conservative continuum), attitudes toward feminism, desire for children, and interest in and ability at sports, and because the two studies on religiosity give opposing results, no particular direction of influence on self-esteem level was expected.

GAY-RELATED ACTIVITIES
AND ATTITUDES

In contrast to the sociodemographic and attitudes and interest variables, considerably more empirical research has addressed the relationship between gay-related activities and attitudes and self-esteem level. The basic premise is that those with high self-esteem may interact with others in ways that differ from those with low levels of self-esteem. In this category the variables explored included self-reports of degree of homosexuality, the age at which one first recognized homosexual feelings, the desire to give up one's sexual orientation, and the feeling that one's sexual orientation is beyond one's control. In addition, social and political involvement with other gay and lesbian individuals, bar attendance, and quantity of sexual activities with other men and women were investigated.

In terms of gay-related activities, there is general agreement on the value of social integration. From their study of gay men, Weinberg and Williams (1974) concluded, "Those higher in social involvement report fewer psychological problems. This was seen as a function of the social psychological support coming from other homosexuals and the effect of this support on self-image" (p. 287). For example, gay men who lived with a gay roommate and were actively involved with gay friends had high levels of self-regard. Socially involved homosexual men anticipated less rejection and discrimination from the heterosexual world. The conception that other, less involved men might have of a universally hostile reaction was replaced by a more realistic appreciation of the complexity of heterosexuals' attitudes and behaviors.

Harry and DeVall (1978) similarly reported that gay men who socialized with gay couples and were socially integrated into the gay community had higher levels of self-esteem than those who were socially isolated. Gay men in another study (Bell & Weinberg, 1978) who were highly involved in the gay subculture had the highest levels of self-acceptance in the sample; lowest scores were achieved by the loners and those frightened to be seen with other gay men. Frequent bar patrons in Chicago were not more or less depressed than others, unless bar attendance was their only source of recreational activities. Such individuals felt more alienated and depressed, had fewer friends and confidants, and had more negative ways of coping with stress (McKirnan & Peterson, 1987b). The fewer the recreational resources, the lower the self-esteem.

Several investigations have reported that gay men low in frequency of sex have similarly low levels of self-acceptance (Reiche & Dannecker, 1977; Weinberg & Williams, 1974). The former study was conducted with a survey questionnaire completed by 789 West German gay men. The authors concluded that although having frequent homosexual sex was unrelated to emotional and mental health, there was a definite relationship between very low levels of homosexual activity and disturbances in self-esteem. Sexually inactive men, they felt, were those who failed to accept their homosexuality.

Contrary to these findings, in a questionnaire study of gay males who were bar patrons, members of homophile organizations, and friends of those who distributed the questionnaire, Harry and DeVall (1978) found self-esteem was unrelated to the number of sex partners. Essentially the same result has been reported by others (Bell & Weinberg, 1978; Weis & Dain, 1979). Low self-esteem characterized both those who had little or no sexual activity and those who had a high number of sexual partners. On the other hand, self-esteem was highest for the relatively monogamous close-coupled and the sexually promiscuous functional categories (Bell & Weinberg, 1978).

Reflecting on their adolescence, the men with high self-esteem in Harry and DeVall's (1978) study tended to define themselves as having been gay at a young age. Unrelated to self-esteem was their degree of heterosexual interest. Weinberg and Williams (1974) reported the same finding: There was little difference in self-acceptance level between bisexual and homosexual males.

Counter to these two studies is other empirical evidence. In Greenberg's (1973) research with 86 members of male homophile organizations, bisexuals who were predominantly heterosexual had significantly lower self-esteem levels than bisexuals predominantly homosexual and those exclusively homosexual. Wayson (1985), however, reported a moderate but nonsignificant trend for bisexual men to have higher self-esteem than either gay or straight volunteers. As acceptance of the self increases after puberty, heterosexual activity should also decrease; Reiche and Dannecker (1977) documented this trend.

Research exploring these issues among lesbians is scant in the psychological and sociological literatures. La Torre and Wendenburg (1983) reported that women with actual sexual experiences with females, regardless of their self-label as straight, bisexual, or lesbian, had higher self-esteem than those without such experiences.

There is more information in regard to attitudes that lesbians and gay males have concerning their sexual orientation. For example, Weinberg and Williams (1974) noted that men committed to their homosexuality and who viewed homosexuality as normal had significantly higher levels of self-acceptance than those who did not share these perspectives. Self-acceptance was highest among individuals who did not anticipate discrimination or worry about exposure, and were either low or high in passing as heterosexual. Low self-acceptance scores were characteristic of those who scored high in anticipating discrimination and exposure of their homosexuality.

In a sample of 190 gay male and lesbian adults (Miranda, 1986), distress at the thought of leading a homosexual life-style and of having same-sex associations was significantly correlated with low self-esteem. Unrelated to self-esteem were the desire for heterosexual or homosexual relationships, sexual arousal, and fantasies of a heterosexual life-style (marriage, love, and family life).

In an interview study (Weinberg, 1983), gay men who accepted their homosexual identity had the highest levels of self-acceptance. In his dissertation, Beebe (1981) reported indirect support for this finding in a metropolitan male sample: Those who accepted their sexual orientation expressed less potential for psychopathology. Of several causal models tested, it was clear that commitment to homosexuality led to positive self-image and psychological adjustment and not the reverse (Hammersmith & Weinberg, 1973). Comparable results were found in a study of gay men in psychiatric clinics and prisons (Schofield, 1965). Without citing empirical data, Miller (1978) agreed with these findings. As "husbands" moved from "trade" (those who engaged in furtive sex and who had a low acceptance of themselves as homosexual) to "faggot" (those with a gay self-identity and who proudly acknowledged this in their life-style), self-esteem increased. Finally, Harry and DeVall (1978) found their Detroit gay men who subscribed to the popular stereotype of homosexuals as shallow, uninteresting, and sick had significantly low levels of self-esteem.

Hypotheses

Several trends emerge from the literature reviewed concerning self-esteem and gay-related activities and interests. There is clear evidence that those involved in the lesbian and gay subcultures, meaning those who participated in gay and lesbian activities and socialized with other lesbians and gays, and who were committed and accepting of their homosexuality, had the highest levels of self-esteem. On the other hand, there is conflicting evidence as to the relationship of self-evaluation and bar attendance, frequency of engaging in homosexual and heterosexual sex, and an individual's stated degree of where he or she is on the heterosexual–homosexual continuum. There is also a suggestion that those who felt their homosexuality at an early age have a positive self-image. All of these relationships are either not documented or poorly investigated among lesbians.

SUPPORT OF FAMILY AND FRIENDS

Weinberg (1983) noted the critical nature of social support for gay men:

> Even after men have labeled themselves as homosexual, they may still have difficulty accepting this self-identity. Acceptance by non-homosexuals may affect the "moral career" of the homosexual both by influencing self-labeling and by helping the individual to develop a positive, self-accepting image of himself as "homosexual, but normal." (p. 215)

The underlying theoretical perspective is reflected appraisals, that is, that an individual's self-image is determined in some measure by the feedback that the individual receives from others in regard to her or his self-worth. Thus, "if one perceives that he is getting good, supportive responses from others, this increases the likelihood that he will have good feelings about himself; and if he perceives that he is being rejected by people who are important to him, he is likely to experience feelings of ambivalence about himself" (Weinberg, 1983, p. 244). For men in his sample, the former had increased levels of comfortableness with their homosexuality, general self-confidence, and self-liking.

In outlining developmental stages of coming out, Coleman (1982) noted that after self-admission comes telling others:

> Acceptance or rejection at this point is critical. Acceptance can have a powerfully positive effect on these individuals. For the first time, they can perceive acceptance for who they are. As a result, positive conceptions of themselves are built and self-esteem increases. (pp. 151–152)

Thus, to be consistent with Weinberg and Coleman, those who are important to a youth's life should have an impact on his or her self-esteem based on whether or not they accept the youth's sexual orientation.

Empirical research has generally supported this model. For example, Weinberg and Williams (1974) reported that gay men who believed that both gays and straights accepted them, were not disgusted by them, and did not worry about exposure, rejection, or discrimination had higher levels of self-acceptance than those who did not share these beliefs. Mature adult lesbians (Raphael & Robinson, 1980) who reported the highest level of self-esteem had the strongest friendship ties but the weakest ties to siblings. Dutch male and female homosexual youths who had high self-esteem generally had more friends and acquaintances (G. Sanders, 1980). But there was little relationship in the Harry and DeVall (1978) study on the measure that reflected the extent to which the respondents had straight friends and self-esteem. "Confidants" represented for McKirnan and Peterson (1987b) not only number of friends but also closeness and dependability (who one would turn to in an emergency). Alienation and negative mood (including low self-esteem) were significantly lower for those who had many confidants.

Hypotheses

It was possible to propose with some confidence that gay and lesbian youths who felt as if they were accepted by family members and friends would have the highest levels of self-esteem. The evidence for the relationship between number of friends and self-evaluation is less certain, but was predicted to be in the same positive direction.

LOVE AND LOVE AFFAIRS

Few correlates of self-esteem have been so extensively investigated as have aspects of love and love relationships. Ponse (1980) emphasized that expressions of warmth and friendship within relationships serve genuine and gratifying needs for the self and for the partner. Thus, various aspects of "love affairs" were explored to determine their relationship with self-esteem level.

Positive self-esteem and self-acceptance were characteristic of gay males who had a long-lasting love relationship, whether with a man (Dickey, 1961; Silverstein, 1981; Weinberg & Williams, 1974; Westmoreland, 1975; Wilkins, 1981) or a woman (Greenberg, 1973; Weinberg & Williams, 1974). Youths from the Netherlands (G. Sanders, 1980) frequently cited living with one partner for life as their ideal life-style for the future. Silverstein (1981) noted that a coupled individual feels "chosen" and so has positive self-esteem.

The nature of the causal linkage is unclear, however. It is equally valid to argue that those with high self-esteem are more likely to stay in a long-term relationship than those with a low opinion of their self-worth. This was the view of Dickey (1961):

The adequate homosexual male, on the other hand, is able to endure the more or less permanent company of another homosexual—especially if the latter also feels self-adequate—and thus is more apt to marry homosexually than is the inadequate male. (p. 121)

Other writers (Bilotta, 1977; Kellogg, 1978) argued that establishing a love relationship is a way of resolving one's gender identity and of reaffirming one's sexual orientation, thus enhancing the sense of completion.

In one study, satisfaction with the "marital" relationship among gay males was best predicted by level of self-esteem, communication, commitment, sexual satisfaction, and family acceptance (Picciotto, 1984). Examining the personality characteristics of 84 gay men, Wilkins (1981) reported that those in ongoing relationships possessed high levels of self-esteem, warmth, and stable affects; those labeled "cruisers" reflected a tendency to be insecure, emotionally labile, and potential sociopaths with impaired superego controls.

Others, however, have registered disagreement with the significant connection between being coupled and high self-esteem. In his dissertation, Wong (1980) found no difference in self-concept level between gay male or lesbian couples and singles. Harry and DeVall (1978) reported that self-esteem among gay men was unrelated to being single, married to a gay man, divorced from a gay man, or coupled with another man for at least a year. In his study of Chicago gay male couples, however, Harry (1984) found that men currently in a love relationship had a modest but significantly higher level of self-esteem than those not in a relationship. He attributed this to the fact that coupledness bears on the affective component of the self-concept. This finding was dependent, however, on the age of the men. Those never in a relationship had lower self-esteem than all others if they were 35 years or older; if under 35 years of age, then the relationship between the two variables was nonsignificant. The younger men may have been a more biased group for testing the relationship between coupledness and self-evaluation because they had not yet had adequate opportunity or time to develop a relationship.

In a extensive study in the San Francisco Bay area, Bell and Weinberg (1978) found that the two highest self-acceptance groups of gay men, equal to the level of the heterosexual men, were the closed-coupleds, the happily marrieds, *and* the functionals, that is, the swinging singles who had little intention of settling into a relationship. Having the lowest level of self-acceptance were two "types" who were clearly not involved with others: the dysfunctionals (the "tormented homosexuals") and the asexuals (the "invisibles"). Legier (1986) extended this research by including lesbians. She, too, found that the unmarried–unsettled women had the poorest psychological adjustment, including a lower level of self-acceptance.

Hypotheses

The results cited above and the findings of Harry (1984) suggest that a more detailed examination of the connection between coupledness and self-esteem is in order. Whether one is in or out of a relationship is too simplistic of a notion to be a good predictor of self-esteem. Thus, although the weight of the empirical literature supports the proposition that those in a love relationship have positive self-esteem, other aspects of love affairs must also be examined. The nature of these other aspects, unfortunately, is seldom specified. The present study included the longevity of the relationship, the age when the first affair began, the sex of the partner, the nature of the first relationship (whether gay or straight), and the number of love affairs, as well as whether the youth currently was in a love affair.

SELF-DESCRIPTIONS AND SELF-WORTH

Researchers have generally not used a lesbian or gay person's self-described personality profile to predict self-esteem level. The exceptions have been studies that focused on the general constructs of masculinity and femininity. This fascination stems, it would appear, from the remnants of equating cross-sexual orientation with cross-gender personality and behavior. These global terms, however, carry particular cultural meanings as to what is feminine and masculine. They may, as well, mask potentially important information that a finer detailed word-by-word analysis of specific personality descriptors would elicit.

The most potent predictor of psychological well-being in several investigations is degree of self-perceived masculinity, for both gay males and lesbians (Carlson & Steuer, 1985; Hooberman, 1979; Siegelman, 1972a; Spence & Helmreich, 1978). Harry (1984) confirmed this pattern for all age groups if the individuals were in a relationship. For those not in a relationship, masculinity predicted self-esteem level for the youngest age groups, but in the oldest group of gay males (45 years or older), femininity predicted positive self-esteem.

Hooberman (1979), studying a group of 37 gay students at the University of Michigan, added the caveat that the acceptance of action-oriented, instrumental sex role attributes best predicted self-esteem level when the more expressive, feminine attributes were not rejected. Thus, androgynous rather than sex-typed students had the highest level of self-esteem.

Green's (1987) confusing findings perhaps best typify the ambiguous research conclusions one can legitimately reach with regard to sex role and self-esteem.

Green reported that his "feminine" males, defined by behavioral measures of gender behavior, scored lower than "masculine" males on the self-satisfaction sub-scale of the Tennessee Self-Concept Scale. He made sense of this finding by noting, "Considering the stigma of having been a 'sissy' or of currently being homosexual, it is not surprising that these men have a less positive self-image" (p. 252). One page later, however, Green reported no significant difference between the two groups on the Adjective Check List scale item self-confidence; the positive correlation was dismissed as an "artifact." The "feminine" males scored higher on the psychological feminine scale of the Adjective Check List (considerate, sensitive, timid, etc.) but not significantly lower on the masculinity scale (aggressive, dominant, self-confident, etc.) than the "masculine" group. On the Bem Sex Role Inventory, however, the two groups did not differ in their distribution across the masculine, feminine, androgynous, and undifferentiated groupings.

Other studies of behavioral measures of femininity and masculinity have essentially yielded few significant differences in predicting self-esteem level (Clingman & Fowler, 1976; Lutz, Roback, & Hart, 1984). There was a slight tendency in the former study for "butch" males and females to score higher on self-confidence than "fem" participants.

Hypotheses

With some trepidation, it was possible to predict that lesbian and gay youth in the present study who described themselves in masculine terms would have the highest level of self-evaluation. For other, non-sex-role descriptors, no hypotheses could be generated.

6

Study Results Predicting Self-Esteem

OVERVIEW

In this chapter the relevant items from the Gay and Lesbian Questionnaire (GAL Q) are described in terms of both the questions and the range of responses available to the participating youths. Results are presented in the following manner. First, descriptive findings are reviewed, consisting of the mean and range of responses for each variable in each cluster, the intercorrelations among these variables, and the correlations of these items with self-esteem. Second, the confirmatory or statistical data analyses are presented. In deciding among the possibilities, a regression analysis using the individual items within a cluster to predict self-esteem was clearly inappropriate because many of the variables within a cluster would naturally be highly intercorrelated. This is not surprising given the rationale (similarity) for forming the clusters. Factor analyses with an oblique rotation transformation were computed on items in each cluster. Factors that had principal components with eigenvalues greater than 1.00 were kept for further analyses. These factors were included in a regression analysis predicting self-esteem.

All analyses are presented separately for lesbians and gay males. Because of the nonrandom manner in which the research procedures were carried out in recruiting participating youths and because of the difficulty in recruiting a lesbian sample, it seemed unwise to assume that gay males and lesbians in the current study were similarly and equally representative of their respective larger populations. It is also important to consider the perspective of several lesbian social scientists who have written on the unique identity development of lesbians as adolescents and as adults.

SOCIODEMOGRAPHIC VARIABLES

Age

The age range was from 14 to 23 years among the gay males and from 16 to 23 years among the lesbians. There were, however, relatively few participating youths at the younger ages (see Chapter 4). Test–retest reliability was 95% agreement; one male celebrated a birthday during the month.

Education

The males completed 8 to 16 years of education; among the females the range was similar, but higher, from 10 to 18 years. Thus, the variability is from junior high school completion to graduate school enrollment. Because the reliability study was conducted during May, the 6 senior subjects increased their educational level by 1 year.

Education × Age

A new category was computed from the education and age variables (ed-age). Two large subdivisions were distinguished: in school and out of school. Chapter 4 indicates the finer distinctions (e.g., high school, college freshman, graduate school) and the definition of each subcategory.

Pubertal Onset

Each youth reported the year when he or she first experienced developing sexually (entering pubescence). The range for males of 6 to 19 years and for females of 8 to 18 years indicates that some youths were unrealistic in their estimation. Although retrospective self-report of pubertal onset is not an ideal procedure to assess pubertal maturation, there is evidence that most individuals are fairly accurate in their assessment (Brooks-Gunn, 1987; Duke, Litt, & Gross, 1980). Test–retest reliability in this study was .90.

Community

In response to the question "Which of the following best describes the community you grew up in?", the youths selected farm, rural area, small town, medium-sized town or suburb, small city or large suburb, or city (usually New York City, Boston, or Chicago). Reliability was .95; one male changed his answer from farm to rural area.

Occupational Status

To assess parental occupational status the youths were asked, "When you were about 12 years old, what was the primary occupation of each of your parents?" The responses were categorized according to Hollingshead's Occupational Status Scale and then grouped into four more inclusive categories: professional (professor, lawyer, business executive, doctor), managerial and lesser professional (accountant, technician, teacher, clergy), sales/clerical (secretary, bank teller, store salesperson), and blue collar (factory worker, farmer, truck driver). One youth changed his father's occupation from store manager to store owner on the retest questionnaire. All maternal occupation answers remained the same.

Descriptive Results for Males

The male youths averaged just over 20 years of age with almost 14 years of education; the average male respondent appeared to be a college sophomore. Pubertal onset was reported on the average to be just before the 12th birthday. The mean occupational status level of their families was lesser professionals, and the mean community size reared in was medium-sized town.

The correlations among the sociodemographic variables and of the sociodemographic variables with self-esteem are presented in Table 6.1. As might be expected, age was highly correlated with education and ed-age. Other correlations were also intuitively sensible: Those most highly educated grew up in suburban and urban areas and in upper class homes, and those with high-status families tended to live in urban areas. Males who reported an early onset of puberty were from the lower occupational status families.

None of the sociodemographic variables was significantly correlated with self-esteem. The highest correlation (.11) was between education and self-esteem level.

Predicting Male Self-Esteem

Three factors were retained for predictive purposes (Table 6.2): Pubertal Onset, consisting of onset of puberty; Age/Education, consisting of age, ed-age, and education; and Hometown Community/Socioeconomic Status, consisting of community size and occupational status. Placed in a regression model (Table 6.3), these factors did not significantly predict the self-esteem of the gay males.

Descriptive Results for Females

The sample of lesbians averaged 20.4 years old and 14.2 years of education. The onset of puberty occurred just before 12 years of age. The mean occupational status of the families was lesser professionals, and the mean community size was a medium-sized town.

Charted in Table 6.4 are the correlations among the five sociodemographic variables and of the sociodemographic variables with self-esteem. Age was significantly related to educational level and with ed-age. Those most likely to be raised in urban areas had higher occupational status families.

Self-esteem level was not significantly correlated with any of the sociodemographic variables. The highest correlations were with community size and educational level.

Predicting Female Self-Esteem

As indicated in Table 6.5, three factors were formed from the sociodemographic variables: Hometown Community/Socioeconomic Status, consisting of

Table 6.1 Correlations among sociodemographic variables and of these variables with self-esteem for males

Variable	Age	Education	Ed-age	Pubertal onset	Hometown community	Parental occupation status	Self-esteem
Age	—	.72**	.49**	.08	.07	.10	.04
Education		—	.30**	.05	.22*	.19*	.11
Ed-age			—	.07	−.01	−.03	.05
Pubertal onset				—	−.04	.20*	.00
Hometown community					—	.23**	.07
Parental occupation status						—	.03
M	20.27	13.85	4.06	11.95	3.76	2.06	22.00
N	214	213	214	204	214	199	212

$*p < .01.$ $**p < .001.$

Table 6.2 Factor solution for sociodemographic variables: Males

Factor	Pubertal Onset	Age/ Education	Hometown Community/ Socioeconomic Status
Pubertal Onset	—	.08	.13
Age/Education		—	.17
Home Community/Socioeconomic Status			—

Variable	Rotated factor pattern[a]		
Age	− .00	.91	.01
Education	− .05	.77	.28
Ed-age	.07	.79	− .27
Pubertal onset	.94	.01	− .06
Hometown community	− .20	.02	.85
Parental occupation status	.41	− .05	.64
Eigenvalue	1.07	1.99	1.23

[a]Standard regression coefficients.

community and occupational status; Age/Education, consisting of age and education; and Pubertal Onset/Educational Class, consisting of onset of puberty and ed-age. These factors did not significantly predict lesbian self-esteem (Table 6.6).

ATTITUDES AND INTERESTS

Religiosity

On a scale of 1 to 9 each youth responded to the question "How religious are you now?" A score of 1 indicated *extremely religious* and a 9 represented *not at all religious*. Test–retest reliability was quite high at .91.

Table 6.3 Regression predicting male self-esteem from sociodemographic factors

Source	Full model				
	df	M^2	F	p	r^2
Model	3	16.55	.61	.61	.01
Error	182	27.10			

Factor	Parameter estimates			
	df	SE	t	p
Pubertal Onset	1	.39	.04	.97
Age/Education	1	.39	1.06	.29
Hometown Community/Socioeconomic Status	1	.40	.63	.53

Note. r^2 denotes proportion of variance of model predicted by the independent variables.

Table 6.4 Correlations among sociodemographic variables and of these variables with self-esteem for females

Variable	Age	Education	Ed-age	Pubertal onset	Hometown community	Parental occupation status	Self-esteem
Age	—	.68**	.52**	−.14	.01	−.12	.04
Education		—	.14	−.11	.08	.02	.14
Ed-age			—	.10	−.12	−.14	−.03
Pubertal onset				—	.13	.12	−.04
Hometown community					—	.19*	.15
Parental occupation status						—	−.00
M	20.39	14.15	4.09	11.87	3.87	2.18	22.30
N	103	103	103	98	103	101	101

*p < .05. ** p < .001.

Political Outlook

In response to the question "How would you describe your political outlook?", the youths indicated their political attitudes on a scale from 1 (*extremely liberal*) to 9 (*extremely conservative*). Reliability of this scale with the subsample youths was .88.

Feminism

Immediately after the global political question was a more specific political question: "How sympathetic do you feel towards the feminist movement?" A score of 1 indicated *extremely sympathetic* and a score of 9 indicated *not at all sympathetic*. Reliability was .82.

Table 6.5 Factor solution for sociodemographic variables: Females

Factor	Hometown Community/ Socioeconomic Status	Age/ Education	Pubertal Onset/ Educational Class
Hometown Community/Socioeconomic Status	—	.08	−.01
Age/Education		—	.08
Pubertal Onset/Educational Class			—

Variable	Rotated factor pattern[a]		
Age	.10	.93	.07
Education	−.23	.87	−.19
Ed-age	.41	.41	.62
Pubertal onset	−.20	−.18	.85
Hometown community	−.74	.17	.05
Parental occupation status	−.72	−.04	.13
Eigenvalue	1.32	1.82	1.16

[a]Standard regression coefficients.

Table 6.6 Regression predicting female self-esteem from sociodemographic factors

Source	df	M^2	Full model F	p	r^2
Model	3	24.34	1.27	.29	.04
Error	90	19.12			

Factor	df	Parameter estimates SE	t	p
Hometown Community/Socioeconomic Status	1	.46	− 1.66	.10
Age/Education	1	.46	1.02	.31
Pubertal Onset/Educational Class	1	.45	− .65	.52

Number of Children Desired

Youths who indicated that at some time in the future they would like to have children, whether biological or adopted, were asked, "How many?" Answers ranged from one to eight or more. Fifteen of 19 youths gave identical responses on the two reliability questionnaires: Ten gave the same number, and five did not want children. Two youths changed their answer from "undecided" to two children, and two youths reversed this on the two questionnaires, from one or two children to "undecided."

Sports

Interest in sports was assessed by the mean score of two questions, "Are you interested in sports and athletic activities?" and "Do you have athletic skills?" The continuum on both scales ranged from 1 to 9, with 1 representing *extreme interest* and *extremely talented*, respectively, and 9 representing *no interest* and *none*, respectively. Test–retest reliabilities were .84 and .87, respectively. The correlations between these two were significant at the .001 level for females (.81) and males (.78) in the full-scale study.

Descriptive Results for Males

The male youths were for the most part not particularly religious or interested in or talented at sports. A larger percentage (18%) said they had no athletic talent than replied that they were extremely talented (8%). The male youths claimed to be fairly liberal and supportive of the feminist movement. Only 3% were "extremely conservatives" (8s or 9s on the 9-point scale), whereas 40% could be classified as "extreme liberals" (1s or 2s). More than one-half (52%) were strong supporters of feminism. Of the 59% of the sample who wanted children, the mean number desired was just under two children.

The correlations among the attitudes and interests variables and of the attitudes and interests variables with self-esteem are presented in Table 6.7. Those who

reported feeling most religious also characterized themselves as politically conservative and not supportive of the feminist movement. As might be expected,
those who were sympathetic to feminism were politically liberal.

The only significant correlation with self-esteem was a liberal political philosophy. All other correlations were quite low.

Predicting Male Self-Esteem

Only one factor was formed from the attitudes and interests variables (Table
6.8). This factor was Liberalism, and its components were political ideology,
feminism, and religiosity (negative correlation). Liberalism did not significantly
predict self-esteem level (Table 6.9).

Descriptive Results for Females

The lesbians were strong supporters of feminism and political liberalism, but
not of religiosity. None of the lesbians could be classified as extremely conservative or nonsympathizers of feminism; at the other end of the spectrum, 61% were
"extreme liberals" and 76% strong supporters of feminism. They considered
themselves to be talented at and interested in sports; 42% reported they were
extremely interested in sports. Of the 65% who desired children, the mean number
wanted was 2.3 children.

Presented in Table 6.10 are the correlations among the attitudes and interests
items and of these items with self-esteem. Politically liberal lesbians were most
sympathetic with the feminist movement and had very little interest in sports.
Liberal politics was negatively correlated with religiosity.

All attitudes and interests items were positively correlated with self-esteem, but
none reached an acceptable level of significance.

Predicting Female Self-Esteem

Two factors emerged from the factor analysis of the attitudes and interests items
(Table 6.11): Liberalism, consisting of political ideology, religiosity (negative cor-

Table 6.7 Correlations among attitudes and interests variables and of these variables with self-esteem for males

Variable	Religiosity	Political outlook	Feminism	Number of children desired	Sports	Self-esteem
Religiosity	—	$-.32**$	$-.20*$	$-.14$	.07	.03
Political outlook		—	$.56**$	.07	$-.11$	$.18*$
Feminism			—	.12	$-.11$	.04
Number of children desired				—	$-.05$	$-.08$
Sports					—	.01
M	6.27	3.19	2.88	1.96	5.25	22.00
N	210	211	211	126	214	212

$*p < .01.$ $**p < .001.$

Table 6.8 Factor solution for attitudes and interests
variables: Males

Factor	Liberalism
Liberalism	1.00

Variable	Rotated factor pattern[a]
Religiosity	.55
Political outlook	− .82
Feminism	− .75
Number of children desired	− .32
Sports	.39
Eigenvalue	1.79

[a]Standard regression coefficients.

Table 6.9 Regression predicting male self-esteem from attitudes and
interests factors

Source	df	M^2	F	p	r^2
		Full model			
Model	1	.14	.01	.94	.00
Error	160	23.06			

Factor	df	SE	t	p
		Parameter estimates		
Liberalism	1	.38	− .08	.94

Table 6.10 Correlations among attitudes and interests variables and of these variables with self-esteem
for females

Variable	Religiosity	Political outlook	Feminism	Number of children desired	Sports	Self-esteem
Religiosity	—	− .23*	− .14	.00	.10	.07
Political outlook		—	.40**	.05	− .32**	.00
Feminism			—	.05	− .23*	.06
Number of children desired				—	− .18	.07
Sports					—	.12
M	6.78	2.39	1.85	2.27	3.94	22.30
N	101	103	101	67	103	101

*p < .05.   **p < .001.

relation), feminism, and sports (negative correlation); and Number of Children, consisting of the number of children desired. The overall regression model predicting self-esteem was not significant (Table 6.12).

GAY-RELATED ACTIVITIES AND ATTITUDES

Sexual Orientation Rating

A modified version of the Kinsey Heterosexual-Homosexual Rating Scale was provided in the GAL Q. Youths indicated on a 7-point continuum their sexual orientation: *exclusively heterosexual, predominantly heterosexual and only slightly homosexual, predominantly heterosexual but significantly homosexual, equally homosexual and heterosexual, predominantly homosexual but significantly heterosexual, predominantly homosexual and only slightly heterosexual,* or *exclusively homosexual.* Test–retest reliability was perfect (1.00).

Table 6.11 Factor solution for attitudes and interests variables: Females

Factor	Liberalism	Number of Children Desired
Liberalism	—	− .11
Number of Children Desired		—
Variable	Rotated factor pattern[a]	
Religiosity	.68	.34
Political outlook	− .78	.05
Feminism	− .65	.02
Number of children desired	.02	.89
Sports	.53	− .37
Eigenvalue	1.77	1.04

[a]Standard regression coefficients.

Table 6.12 Regression predicting female self-esteem from attitudes and interests factors

Source	df	M^2	F	p	r^2
			Full model		
Model	2	15.92	.64	.53	.02
Error	62	25.01			

Factor	df	SE	t	p
		Parameter estimates		
Liberalism	1	.63	.62	.54
Number of Children Desired	1	.62	− .87	.39

Age of First Homosexual Feelings

The age at which a youth first remembered having homosexual feelings was probed. Responses were then grouped into six categories: infancy (0 to 2 years), preschool (3 to 6 years), childhood (7 to 11 years), early adolescence (12 to 14 years), middle adolescence (15 to 17 years), and late adolescence (18 years or older). Agreement on this age was quite high (.96) over the course of a month with the reliability sample.

Give Up Homosexuality

Two statements assessed the degree to which respondents were committed to their homosexuality: "I would not give up my homosexuality even if I could" and "I feel my life would be much easier if I were heterosexual." Youths scored each statement on a 1 to 9 continuum, from *strongly agree* to *strongly disagree*. Scores on the second statement were reversed, added to the first, and divided by two. A high score indicates a desire to give up one's homosexuality. Reliabilities on these two questions were .45 and .85, respectively. In the study's data set the two items significantly correlated ($p < .001$) with each other among females (.43) and males (.32).

Beyond Control

On the same 1 to 9 scale each youth responded to two statements that addressed whether an individual could choose her or his sexual orientation: "Being homosexual is a conscious choice I have made" and "Being homosexual is something that is completely beyond one's control." Scores on the second were reversed, added to the first, and divided by two. A high score indicates that a youth felt he or she had no choice in being lesbian/gay; a low score implies a conviction that sexual orientation is under one's control. Reliability coefficients were quite high (.78 and .88, respectively) for both items. The two were significantly ($p < .001$) correlated with each other for females (.40) and males (.39) in the primary study.

Gay Rights

Each youth was asked, "How active have you been in the gay rights movement?" Responses varied on a 9-point scale from *extremely active* to *not at all active*. Test–retest reliability was .87.

Gay Bar

Nine categories were given for the question "How often do you go to gay bars or clubs?" These ranged from *daily* to *never*. Reliability over the course of a month was .83.

Gay and Lesbian Socialization

The same categories were also applied to the question "Excluding bars, how often do you go to public places where gay men and/or lesbians socialize, such as a coffeehouse, gay or lesbian center, dance, etc.?" Reliability on this question was .92.

Gay and Lesbian Activities

On a 9-point scale from *extremely involved* to *not at all involved*, the youths marked their response to the question "During the last year how involved have you been in any organized gay male and lesbian activities?" The test–retest correlation was .80.

Periodicals

Each participant was asked how many gay periodicals she or he read or subscribed to on a regular basis. Categories were *none, one, two, three*, and *four or more*. Test–retest reliability was nearly perfect (.99).

Male and Female Sex Partners

Each youth was requested to state the number of his or her sexual relations, separately for each sex. Nine response categories were given: *0, 1, 2, 3–5, 6–10, 11–20, 21–50, 51–100*, and *101 +*. Reliability coefficient was .98 for male and .95 for female partners.

Descriptive Results for Males

The male youths were predominantly homosexual, averaging 6.2 on the 7-point scale (Table 6.13). Many felt their homosexual tendencies at a relatively early age; the mean was the category 7 to 11 years of age, with 19% of the sample knowing prior to 6 years of age. Congruent with these two results (exclusively homosexual and felt homosexuality at an early age), the gay youths were at the extreme (7.03) end of the 9-point scale in terms of feeling that their sexual orientation was beyond their control. The participants were at the midpoint in terms of feeling that they would give up their homosexuality if they could and feeling that life would be easier if they were heterosexual.

The male youths on the average were somewhat inactive in the gay rights movement (36% replied that they never participated). Similarly, many were inactive in organized gay and lesbian activities and socialization with other lesbians and gays in public places. Almost one-half went to a gay activity only once a year or less. But in terms of bar attendance, more than one-third went weekly. The average was going to a gay bar once a month. The gay males on the average regularly read one gay periodical, although more than one-half read none. Forty-six percent of the male youths were heterosexual virgins; 5% had never experienced homosexual sex. High frequency of sex was relatively rare: 10% had more

Table 6.13 Correlations among gay-related activities and attitudes variables and of these variables with self-esteem for males

Variable	Sexual orientation	Age first felt homosexual	Give up desire	Beyond control	Gay rights	Gay bars	Gay/ Lesbian socialization	Gay/ Lesbian activities	Periodicals	Sex partners		Self- esteem
										Number male	Number female	
Sexual orientation	—	-.27***	-.16**	.42***	.27***	.27***	.22***	.34***	.26***	.20**	-.36***	.17**
Age first felt homosexual		—	.10	-.18**	-.25***	-.15*	-.12	-.28***	-.17**	-.17**	.00	.01
Give up			—	-.05	-.34***	-.07	-.32***	-.35***	-.17**	.00	.01	-.26***
Beyond control				—	.15*	-.03	.09	.19**	.01	-.11	-.22**	.01
Gay rights					—	.18**	.45***	.76***	.39***	.14*	-.04	.14*
Gay bars						—	.22**	.18**	.17**	.42***	-.01	.03
Gay/lesbian socialization							—	.59***	.37***	.15*	-.10	.02
Gay/lesbian activities								—	.42***	.17**	-.08	.09
Periodicals									—	.20**	-.06	.01
Sex partners												
Number male										—	.16*	.09
Number female											—	.03
M	6.28	3.30	4.40	7.03	5.88	4.61	4.73	5.65	1.89	5.33	2.26	22.00
N	213	208	207	204	214	214	212	212	213	212	213	212

*p < .05.   **p < .01.   ***p < .001.

than 50 male partners and less than 1% had over 50 female partners. The mean number of sexual relations was with 6 to 10 men and 1 woman.

The 11 activity variables and their correlations with each other and with self-esteem are presented in Table 6.13. Many of the correlations were quite high, such as between gay rights and gay activities (.76) and gay socialization and gay activities (.59). The highest correlates of positive self-esteem were having little desire to give up one's homosexuality, reporting exclusive homosexuality, and being actively involved in gay rights. Overall, however, relatively few of the variables were significantly related to self-esteem level.

Predicting Male Self-Esteem

Four factors emerged from factor analysis of the gay-related activities and attitudes variables (Table 6.14). These were Heterosexual Acts, which consisted of the number of females variable; Activism, which comprised gay/lesbian activities, gay rights, gay/lesbian socialization, and give up desire (negative correlation); Always Gay, which comprised the feel homosexual at young age and beyond control variables; and Gay Bar/Sex, which comprised the gay bar and number of males variables. The overall self-esteem regression model was not significantly predicted from these factors (Table 6.15).

Descriptive Results for Females

On the average, the lesbian sample rated themselves a 5.8 on the 7-point heterosexual to homosexual continuum and felt their sexual orientation for the first time during early adolescence (12 to 14 years of age) (Table 6.16). Relatively few (10%) reported recognition of homosexual feelings before age 6 years; an equal number (11%) waited until they were 18 years or older. The lesbian youths generally believed they would not give up their sexual orientation even if they could (one point below the mean scale item on the give up desire variable) and that their homosexuality was beyond their control (one point above the mean scale item on the beyond control variable).

As a sample, the lesbians were only moderately active in the gay rights movement and in organized lesbian activities. Forty-five percent went to a lesbian or gay event once a year or less. An average lesbian youth went to a lesbian bar two to three times per month (28% went weekly), publicly socialized with other lesbians and gays once a month (19% once a year or less), and regularly read one lesbian periodical (more than two-thirds read none).

The average lesbian had the same number of male and female sexual partners, two to three during her childhood and adolescence. Twelve percent were homosexually virgin, and 19% heterosexually virgin. Less than 1% of the sample had more than 50 sexual partners, of either sex.

The correlations among the 11 lesbian activities variables and of those with self-esteem are presented in Table 6.16. Lesbian activities was highly correlated with gay rights (.68) and socialization (.61). Only one variable, feeling lesbian at a young age, was significantly correlated with self-esteem.

Table 6.14 Factor solution for gay-related activities and attitudes variables: Males

Factor	Heterosexual Acts	Activism	Always Gay	Gay Bar/ Sex
Heterosexual Acts	—	.15	−.22	−.06
Activism		—	−.28	.26
Always Gay			—	−.10
Gay Bar/Sex				—

Variable	Rotated factor pattern[a]			
Sexual orientation	−.50	−.04	.50	−.28
Age first felt homosexual	−.32	.06	−.75	.15
Give up desire	−.03	.60	−.00	−.17
Beyond control	−.18	.04	.73	.26
Gay rights	.13	−.83	.13	.06
Gay bars	−.16	.03	−.05	−.82
Gay/lesbian socialization	−.13	−.79	−.21	−.04
Gay/lesbian activities	.03	−.86	.12	.02
Periodicals	−.12	−.55	−.16	−.26
Sex partners				
Number male	.22	.01	.05	−.79
Number female	.90	−.02	.06	−:05
Eigenvalue	1.21	2.31	1.28	1.45

[a]Standard regression coefficients.

Predicting Female Self-Esteem

Five primary factors emerged from the factor analysis of the gay-related activities and attitudes variables (Table 6.17): Lesbian Bar/Sex, consisting of the number of females and lesbian bar variables; Heterosexual Acts, which consisted of the number of males variable; Recently Lesbian, comprising the feel homosexual at young age and beyond control variables (both negative correlations); Activism, comprising the gay/lesbian activities, gay rights, and gay/lesbian socialization

Table 6.15 Regression predicting male self-esteem from gay-related activities and attitudes factors

Source	Full model				
	df	M^2	F	p	r^2
Model	4	22.76	.90	.47	.02
Error	188	25.39			

Factor	Parameter estimates			
	df	SE	t	p
Heterosexual Acts	1	.38	.32	.75
Activism	1	.39	1.57	.12
Always Gay	1	.39	.52	.60
Gay Bar/Sex	1	.38	.02	.99

Table 6.16 Correlations among gay-related activities and attitudes variables and of these variables with self-esteem for females

Variable	Sexual orientation	Age first felt homosexual	Give up desire	Beyond control	Gay rights	Lesbian bars	Lesbian/Gay socialization	Lesbian/Gay activities	Periodicals	Sex partners		Self-esteem
										Number male	Number female	
Sexual orientation	—	-.20*	-.14	.13	.36***	.13	.08	.29**	.29**	-.29**	.35***	-.01
Age first felt homosexual		—	.12	-.15	-.08	-.03	-.10	-.06	-.25***	.11	-.22*	-.24*
Give up desire			—	.10	-.14	.05	-.16	-.10	-.19	-.04	.00	-.10
Beyond control				—	.21*	.07	.11	.27**	-.03	-.02	-.11	.09
Gay rights					—	.04	.43***	.68***	.26**	-.15	.04	.05
Lesbian bars						—	.03	.01	.01	-.09	.38***	.09
Lesbian/gay socialization							—	.61***	.20*	.04	-.05	-.15
Lesbian/gay activities								—	.28**	.00	.01	.07
Periodicals									—	-.14	.02	.07
Sex partners												
Number male										—	.05	-.11
Number female											—	.07
M	5.76	3.99	3.67	5.32	5.51	4.37	4.77	5.56	1.52	3.58	3.45	22.30
N	101	101	100	101	103	103	103	103	103	102	103	101

$*p < .05$ $**p < .01.$ $***p < .001.$

81

variables; and Give Up Desire, which consisted of the give up desire variable. The overall regression model based on these five factors predicting self-esteem was not significant (Table 6.18).

Table 6.17 Factor solution for gay-related activities and attitudes variables: Females

Factor	Lesbian Bar/Sex	Heterosexual Acts	Recently Lesbian	Activism	Give Up Desire
Lesbian Bar/Sex	—	−.13	−.15	−.05	−.03
Heterosexual Acts		—	.18	.14	.08
Recently Lesbian			—	.22	.08
Activism				—	.16
Give Up Desire					—
Variable	Rotated factor pattern[a]				
Sexual orientation	.44	−.44	−.10	−.27	−.16
Age first felt homosexual	−.15	−.04	.79	−.20	.30
Give up desire	.04	−.12	−.02	.02	.79
Beyond control	−.19	.02	−.74	−.20	.47
Gay rights	.02	−.20	.06	−.81	−.04
Lesbian bars	.67	−.02	.05	−.06	.38
Lesbian/gay socialization	−.08	.29	.01	−.76	−.07
Lesbian/gay activities	.01	.07	−.00	−.92	.06
Periodicals	−.00	−.26	−.21	−.21	−.44
Sexual partners					
Number male	.11	.93	−.05	−.07	−.07
Number female	.90	.14	−.01	.07	−.08
Eigenvalue	1.48	1.22	1.14	2.12	1.28

[a]Standard regression coefficients.

Table 6.18 Regression predicting female self-esteem from gay-related activities and attitudes factors

Source	df	M^2	F	p	r^2
	Full model				
Model	5	22.29	1.09	.37	.06
Error	89	20.54			

Factor	df	SE	t	p
	Parameter estimates			
Lesbian Bar/Sex	1	.48	.48	.63
Heterosexual Acts	1	.49	−.69	.49
Recently Lesbian	1	.49	−1.88	.06
Activism	1	.48	−.75	.45
Give Up Desire	1	.48	−.30	.76

SUPPORT OF FAMILY AND FRIENDS

Measures

To assess acceptance from various sources, each participant responded to the GAL Q question "How has each of the following persons reacted (or how do you think they would react) to the fact that you are lesbian/gay?" The person categories included mother, father, closest sibling, best heterosexual female friend, best heterosexual male friend, and closest academic advisor/professor. The four levels of responses were *accepting (or it would not matter)*, *tolerant (but not accepting)*, *intolerant (but not rejecting)*, and *rejecting*. Reliability coefficients ranged from .58 for mother and father and .67 for sibling to 1.00 for female friend, .96 for male friend, and .95 for academic advisor.

Further evidence of support, from friends, was assessed by the question "Excluding relatives, how many close friends do you have?" The six categories were gay men, lesbians, bisexual men, bisexual women, heterosexual men, and heterosexual women. Because many of the responses were general descriptors, for example, *lots* or *several*, four categories were created: (a) none; (b) few, several, one to three; (c) four to six; and (d) lots, many, seven or more. Test–retest reliabilities for these categories were .75, .81, .57, .64, .94, and .71 for gay men, lesbians, bisexual men, bisexual women, heterosexual men, and heterosexual women, respectively.

Descriptive Results for Males

Gay males reported feeling the greatest acceptance from their best heterosexual female and male friends (Table 6.19). Perceived acceptance was relatively poor from father and mother; less than one-quarter reported full acceptance from the father, and one-third reported full acceptance from the mother. The percentages were three times higher for the best heterosexual friends; full acceptance from sibling (58%) and academic advisor (62%) was somewhat lower.

The youths reported having many gay (32%) and heterosexual female (33%) friends. Heterosexual male friends were lower in number than these two primarily because very few gay males reported that they had "many" straight male friends. Eight to nine percent of the youths reported that they had no friends who were gay, heterosexual female, or heterosexual male. Not only were bisexual friends rare (nearly 60% said they had none), but relatively few (9%) of the gay males had "many" lesbian friends. Overall, gay males reported a greater number of male than female friends, regardless of the sexual orientation of the friends.

Table 6.19 presents the correlations among the support variables and their relationship with self-esteem for the study's males. Most striking were the nearly uniform significant correlations among the perceptions of the males that if their homosexuality was accepted (or would be if the person knew his sexual orientation) by one family member, a peer friend, or an academic advisor then they would be accepted by the others. The correlations were particularly high between the parents and among male friend, female friend, and academic advisor. These variables, in turn, were generally not highly correlated with the number of friends reported by the male youths. The lone exception was gay males who felt accepted by a heterosexual female friend or an academic advisor; such individuals reported

Table 6.19 Correlations among support of family and friends variables and of these variables with self-esteem for males

Variable	Mother	Father	Sibling	Female friend	Male friend	Professor	Gay friend	Lesbian friend	Bisexual male friend	Bisexual female friend	Heterosexual male friend	Heterosexual female friend	Self-esteem
Mother	—												.14*
Father	.52***	—											.11
Sibling	.41***	.28***	—										.13
Female friend	.21**	.25***	.29***	—									.19**
Male friend	.23**	.30***	.21**	.67***	—								.30***
Professor	.19*	.16	.20*	.59***	.62***	—							.22**
Gay friend	-.05	-.05	.03	.19**	.07	.15	—						.10
Lesbian friend	.02	.02	.04	.19**	.14	.19*	.34***	—					.12
Bisexual male friend	-.06	-.11	-.05	.04	-.09	.19*	.05	.24***	—				.03
Bisexual female friend	-.03	-.06	-.03	.09	-.00	.18*	.06	.25***	.76***	—			.01
Heterosexual male friend	.04	.12	.04	.06	.03	.12	.30***	.27***	.31***	.23**	—		.14*
Heterosexual female friend	.02	.07	.05	.14	.06	.06	.33***	.34***	.22**	.26***	.67***	—	.14*
M	1.94	1.56	2.33	2.72	2.52	2.38	2.83	1.94	2.12	2.09	2.57	2.81	22.00
N	207	200	198	200	187	136	202	195	183	182	197	201	212

*p < .05. **p < .01. ***p < .001.

a high number of gay, lesbian, bisexual male, and bisexual female friends (academic advisor only).

Males who reported a large number of friends in any particular sex or sexual orientation group also reported a large number of friends in the other groups. In general, sexual orientation appeared to be a better predictor than sex or friendship number. The correlations within a sexual orientation group (i.e., gay male-lesbian, bisexual male–bisexual female, heterosexual male–heterosexual female) averaged higher (.59) than across sexual orientation groups (.24), same-sex friends (.26), and other sex friends (.35).

Gay males who felt accepted by a heterosexual male or female best friend, an academic advisor, or their mother or who had a large number of heterosexual friends had the highest levels of self-esteem. Most striking was the significance level ($p < .0001$) of the correlation between acceptance by heterosexual male best friend and positive self-esteem.

Predicting Male Self-Esteem

Table 6.20 presents the four support factors for the gay males: Straight/Gay Friends, which included the straight female friends, straight male friends, gay friends, and lesbian friends variables; Bisexual Friends, which included the bisexual male friends and bisexual female friends variables; Mother/Sibling Accept, which included the mother accepts and sibling accepts variables; and Friends Accept, which included the male friend accepts, advisor accepts, and female friend accepts variables. These factors did not predict the self-esteem level of the male sample (Table 6.21).

Descriptive Results for Females

Lesbian youths felt the highest acceptance levels from heterosexual female and male friends and an academic advisor (Table 6.22). Less than 5% felt rejection from these individuals. Perceived acceptance from parents was relatively low; only one-quarter felt acceptance from their parents, and one-fifth felt rejection. Acceptance from siblings was more similar to that of friends than that of parents (10% felt rejection).

The youths reported many lesbian (31%) and heterosexual female (34%) friends. Only 1% had no heterosexual female friends. Relatively few lesbians (11%) had "lots" of gay friends, one-half of the number who reported they had no gay friends. Relatively few had bisexual male friends; two-thirds said they had none. Disregarding the sexual orientation of the friends, lesbians reported strikingly more female than male friends.

Table 6.22 presents the correlations among the various support variables and of the support variables with self-esteem. Lesbians who felt acceptance from one parent also felt acceptance from the other parent, a sibling, and a heterosexual male best friend. In addition, youths who reported acceptance from their father also reported acceptance from their academic advisor; acceptance from heterosexual male best friend was significantly correlated with acceptance from heterosexual female best friend and academic advisor. Acceptance from father, sibling,

Table 6.20   Factor solution for support variables: Males

Factor	Straight/Gay Friends	Bisexual Friends	Mother/Sibling Accept	Friends Accept
Straight/Gay Friends	—	.19	−.13	−.19
Bisexual Friends		—	.06	−.14
Mother/Sibling Accept			—	.37
Friends Accept				—

Variable	Rotated factor pattern[a]			
Mother	−.00	.02	.85	.04
Father	−.13	.32	.40	.28
Sibling	.02	−.11	.84	−.09
Female friend	−.04	.01	.10	.84
Male friend	.02	.06	−.09	.96
Professor	.05	−.15	−.01	.85
Gay friend	.73	.05	.01	−.08
Lesbian friend	.73	.04	.14	−.16
Bisexual male friend	.04	.87	.07	−.06
Bisexual female friend	−.01	.86	−.14	.02
Heterosexual male friend	.80	−.06	.03	.05
Heterosexual female friend	.82	.02	−.11	.17
Eigenvalue	2.24	1.53	1.42	2.06

[a]Standard regression coefficients.

heterosexual male friend, and academic advisor was negatively correlated with having a best heterosexual female friend.

Lesbians who reported they had many gay friends also had many lesbian, bisexual female, and bisexual male friends; if they had many lesbian friends, then they had many bisexual and heterosexual female friends as well. Number of bisexual male and number of bisexual female friends were positively correlated with each other; number of heterosexual male and number of heterosexual female friends, with each other. The correlations within sexual orientation group were quite high

Table 6.21   Regression predicting male self-esteem from support factors

Source	df	M^2	F	p	r^2
		Full model			
Model	4	34.02	1.22	.31	.05
Error	84	27.93			

Factor	df	SE	t	p
	Parameter estimates			
Straight/Gay Friends	1	.58	−.46	.65
Bisexual Friends	1	.58	.78	.44
Mother/Sibling Accept	1	.61	.73	.46
Friends Accept	1	.62	1.48	.14

Table 6.22 Correlations among support of family and friends variables and of these variables with self-esteem for females

Variable	Mother	Father	Sibling	Female friend	Male friend	Professor	Gay friend	Lesbian friend	Bisexual male friend	Bisexual female friend	Heterosexual male friend	Heterosexual female friend	Self-esteem
Mother	—	.33***	.30**	.13	.26*	.12	-.08	-.09	.06	.04	-.02	-.02	.07
Father		—	.38***	.13	.38***	.25*	.03	-.06	.21	.11	-.14	-.29**	.14
Sibling			—	-.12	.13	.10	-.01	.03	-.04	-.03	-.08	-.22*	.10
Female friend				—	.38***	.17	-.02	.06	.05	.09	-.01	.08	.08
Male friend					—	.25*	.01	-.03	.12	.11	-.14	-.24*	-.08
Professor						—	.06	-.10	.11	.09	-.05	-.22	.20
Gay friend							—	.44***	.31**	.34***	.19	.10	-.21*
Lesbian friend								—	.10	.21*	.11	.24*	-.06
Bisexual male friend									—	.76***	.15	.20	.22*
Bisexual female friend										—	.06	.15	.08
Heterosexual male friend											—	.63***	.11
Heterosexual female friend												—	.15
M	1.72	1.64	2.32	2.66	2.61	2.53	2.22	2.93	1.83	2.30	2.42	2.90	22.30
N	101	96	96	102	85	75	93	94	87	94	92	97	101

*p < .05. **p < .01. ***p < .001.

(average = .61), greater than with other sexual orientation groups (.18), same-sex peers (.21), and other-sex peers (.30).

Few of the support variables significantly predicted the self-esteem level of the female youths. Those with high self-esteem had many bisexual male friends but few gay friends; however, these correlations were marginally significant.

Predicting Female Self-Esteem

The support variables formed four factors (Table 6.23): Lesbian/Gay Friends, which comprised the lesbian friends and gay friends variables; Bisexual Friends, which comprised the bisexual male friends and bisexual female friends variables; Female Friend Accepts, which constituted the female friend accepts variable; and Family Accepts, which included the father accepts, sibling accepts, mother accepts, and male friend accepts variables. Self-esteem scores among the lesbians were significantly predicted by the support factors (Table 6.24). A large number of bisexual friends was the single best predictor of lesbian self-esteem. The Family Accepts factor approached significance.

LOVE AND LOVE AFFAIRS

Measures

The first question that assessed love affairs on the GAL Q was "Have you had a meaningful love affair?" If the answer was "yes," then youths were asked to list

Table 6.23 Factor solutions for support variables: Females

Factor	Lesbian/Gay Friends	Bisexual Friends	Female Friend Accepts	Family Accepts
Lesbian/Gay Friends	—	.15	−.01	.14
Bisexual Friends		—	−.10	.03
Female Friend Accepts			—	.10
Family Accepts				—

Variable	Rotated factor pattern[a]			
Mother	−.25	−.15	−.19	.63
Father	.02	−.23	−.03	.81
Sibling	−.16	.10	−.36	.74
Female friend	−.13	−.04	.88	−.07
Male friend	−.07	.02	.22	.60
Professor	.20	−.08	.36	.46
Gay friend	.66	.05	−.15	−.17
Lesbian friend	.80	−.26	−.13	−.04
Bisexual male friend	−.14	.96	.00	−.10
Bisexual female friend	−.02	.83	−.15	.01
Heterosexual male friend	.39	.43	.24	.29
Heterosexual female friend	.40	.36	.14	.53
Eigenvalue	1.48	2.03	1.23	2.50

[a]Standard regression coefficients.

Table 6.24 Regression predicting female self-esteem from support factors

			Full model		
Source	df	M^2	F	p	r^2
Model	4	49.51	2.98	.03	.23
Error	39	16.59			

		Parameter estimates		
Factor	df	SE	t	p
Lesbian/Gay Friends	1	.66	.10	.92
Bisexual Friends	1	.63	3.17	.00
Female Friend Accepts	1	.62	− .43	.67
Family Accepts	1	.70	1.55	.13

all affairs, including the sex of the person, when it began, and how long it lasted. The number of love affairs ranged from none to eight. The second category was the presence or absence of a current love affair. Longevity, the average length of all love affairs, was determined by dividing length of all relationships by the number of love affairs.

The fourth and fifth love affairs variables investigated were the age when the first love affair occurred and the sex of the person involved. Finally, the percentage of homosexual love affairs was determined. Thus there were six love variables in all.

There were several changes in reports of love affairs between the first and second administration of the reliability questionnaire. There were no changes in whether the individual had experienced a meaningful love relationship or the sex of the other person. One male had a new current affair and another male's new current love affair was a previous love affair. Four youths added love affairs they had neglected to mention at Time 1; two of these were a first love affair during their adolescence. Two youths added 6 months to a past relationship's longevity, and one male added a year to his age when his first relationship began. On the whole, however, the stability of love relationships self-reports was quite striking.

Descriptive Results for Males

The gay males averaged 1.4 love affairs; one-half had been involved in either one or two self-defined love affairs at the time of data collection (Table 6.25). One-third had never had a love affair, and 41% were in a current relationship. Love affairs lasted on the average just under 1 year, ranging from several days to 7 years. Of all love affairs, 58% were with other males. Of those who had at least one love affair, the age of the first love affair was 17.2 years. The first love affair was more likely to be with a male than with a female.

Table 6.25 presents the correlations among the love affair variables and of those variables with self-esteem. Males who had many love affairs were most likely to be involved in a love affair at data collection, but the average length of their

Table 6.25 Correlations among love affairs variables and of these variables with self-esteem for males

Variable	Number of love affairs	Current affair	Longevity	Age of first affair	Sex of first lover	Percentage of gay affairs	Self-esteem
Number of love affairs	—	.44***	−.20*	−.35***	−.22*	.40***	.18**
Current affair		—	.11	−.12	−.03	.49***	.17**
Longevity			—	−.44***	−.07	.04	−.04
Age of first affair				—	.12	.06	−.03
Sex of first lover					—	.82***	.17
Percentage of gay affairs						—	.16*
M	1.40	1.57	51.03	17.17	1.69	.58	22.00
N	208	204	141	108	108	208	212

*p < .05.   **p < .01.   ***p < .001.

relationships was relatively short. Such men also tended to have had their first sexual encounter with a female and at a young age, but subsequent love affairs were more likely to be homosexual than heterosexual.

Those currently in a love affair were also likely to have a large percentage of their total love affairs being homosexual. In addition, youths who had their first sexual encounter with a male were more likely ($r = .82$) to have a high percentage of homosexual love affairs than those whose first sexual encounter was with a female. Finally, those who began love affairs at an early age were most likely to have long-term love affairs.

Gay males with the highest level of self-esteem reported many love affairs, a current love affair, and a large percentage of homosexual affairs.

Predicting Male Self-Esteem

Three factors emerged from the factor analysis of the love affair variables (Table 6.26): Affair Length, consisting of the longevity of affairs and young first age of affair variables; Gay Affairs, consisting of the percentage of gay affairs and homosexual first affair variables; and Affair Number, consisting of the number of love affairs and current affair variables. The regression model predicting self-esteem was significant (Table 6.27). The factors that most contributed were Affair Number and Gay Affairs.

Descriptive Results for Females

The lesbian youths averaged 2.4 love affairs; 14% reported that they have never had a relationship and 11% have had five or more. Sixty-seven percent of the youths were in a love affair at the time of data collection (Table 6.28). Love affairs lasted an average of 15 months, with a range of a few days to just under 10 years. The first love affair was equally likely to be with another female as with a male and occurred at 16.6 years of age. The majority (61%) of all love affairs were with other women.

The correlations among the love affair variables and of those variables with self-esteem are presented in Table 6.28. Lesbians who experienced a love affair at

Table 6.26 Factor solution for love affairs variables: Males

Factor	Affair Length	Gay Affairs	Affair Number
Affair Length	—	− .09	.10
Gay Affairs		—	− .14
Affair Number			—

Variable	Rotated factor pattern[a]		
Number of love affairs	.00	− .15	.84
Current affair	.05	− .15	− .81
Longevity	.89	− .00	− .24
Age of first affair	− .79	− .01	− .32
Sex of first lover	− .03	.94	− .02
Percentage of affairs	.03	.96	.02
Eigenvalue	1.41	1.81	1.48

[a]Standard regression coefficients.

a young age were most likely to have had many love affairs, to be involved in a current love affair, and to have had love affairs that lasted a long time. If a lesbian's love affairs were predominantly homosexual rather than heterosexual then she was more likely to have a current love affair, to have shorter love affairs, and to have had her first love affair with another female ($r = .79$). Finally, a lesbian with many love affairs was likely to be currently involved in one.

None of the love affair variables was significantly correlated with self-esteem. Those youths who were in a current affair ($p < .12$) and who had love affairs that lasted a long time ($p < .11$) tended to have high self-esteem.

Predicting Female Self-Esteem

The love affair variables formed three factors (Table 6.29): Lesbian Affairs, comprising the percentage of lesbian affairs and homosexual first affair variables;

Table 6.27 Regression predicting male self-esteem from love affairs factors

Source	df	M^2	F	p	r^2
		Full model			
Model	3	83.65	3.54	.02	.09
Error	104	23.66			

Factor	df	SE	t	p
		Parameter estimates		
Affair Length	1	.47	− .21	.84
Gay Affairs	1	.48	2.12	.04
Affair Number	1	.48	2.73	.008

Table 6.28 Correlations among love affairs variables and of these variables with self-esteem for females

Variable	Number of love affairs	Current affair	Longevity	Age of first affair	Sex of first lover	Percentage of lesbian affairs	Self-esteem
Number of love affairs	—	.44***	−.20	−.42***	.04	.16	.10
Current affair		—	−.00	−.22*	.05	.31**	.16
Longevity			—	−.36***	.17	−.23*	.17
Age of first affair				—	−.07	−.01	−.02
Sex of first lover					—	.79***	−.05
Percentage of lesbian affairs						—	.05
M	2.35	1.33	65.91	16.64	1.56	.61	22.30
N	99	98	89	78	79	99	101

*p < .05.   **p < .01.   ***p < .001.

Affair Length, comprising the longevity of affairs and young first age of affair variables; and Affair Number, comprising the number of love affairs and current affair variables. The three factors did not significantly predict level of lesbian self-esteem (Table 6.30).

SELF-DESCRIPTIONS AND SELF-WORTH

Measures

Included in the GAL Q was a list of 17 self-descriptive words or phrases used by Blumstein and Schwartz (1983) as a means to assess one's view of the self. Each youth rated himself or herself on a 9-point scale from *extremely* to *not at all* descriptive on the following dimensions (test–retest reliability coefficients in pa-

Table 6.29 Factor solution for love affairs variables: Females

Factor	Lesbian Affairs	Affair Length	Affair Number
Lesbian Affairs	—	−.12	−.01
Affair Length		—	.09
Affair Number			—
Variable	Rotated factor pattern[a]		
Number of love affairs	−.05	−.05	.87
Current affair	−.00	.13	−.77
Longevity	−.05	.90	−.25
Age of first affair	−.09	−.70	−.52
Sex of first lover	−.94	.04	.05
Percentage of lesbian affairs	.95	.02	.02
Eigenvalue	1.77	1.30	1.66

[a]Standard regression coefficients.

Table 6.30 Regression predicting female self-esteem from love affairs factors

Source	df		Full model		
		M^2	F	p	r^2
Model	3	6.38	.36	.78	.01
Error	73	17.71			

Factor	df	Parameter estimates		
		SE	t	p
Lesbian Affairs	1	.48	−.76	.45
Affair Length	1	.49	.56	.58
Affair Number	1	.48	.21	.83

rentheses): "accomplished in my chosen field" (.68), "muscular build" (.89), "compassionate" (.65), "outgoing" (.78), "aggressive" (.88), "express tender feelings easily" (.64), "forceful" (.69), "sexy looking" (.58), "affectionate" (.56), "competitive with others" (.84), "shy" (.75), "self-sufficient" (.67), "ambitious" (.82), "romantic" (.92), "athletic" (.92), "understanding of others" (.49), and "movie star good looking" (.78).

To assess the important dimensions of lesbian and gay sense of self-worth, I developed a list of 12 items that were included in the GAL Q. Youths rated on a 9-point scale how important the following were for their sense of self-worth (test–retest reliability coefficients in parentheses): "career" (present/future) (.78), "being in a lover relationship" (.38), "having children" (.88), "an active social life" (.81), "frequency of having sex" (.75), "close female friends" (.72), "physical looks" (.90), "academic success" (.64), "close male friends" (.72), "relationship with parents" (.86), "religion" (.93), and "material possessions" (.87).

Descriptive Results for Males

The gay males were most likely to describe themselves as romantic, understanding, compassionate, affectionate, and ambitious and least likely to attribute to themselves movie star good looks, athletic abilities, shy, and muscular build. All adjectives but the last of the most characteristic group are of the "expressive" or feminine variety, whereas three of the least frequent self-descriptors are typically attributed to masculinity.

The correlations among the 17 self-description adjectives and of those adjectives with self-esteem are presented in Table 6.31. A number of clusters are apparent from the correlations among the adjectives. These will be pursued more systematically in the factor analysis presented below. The highest correlations were between being affectionate and expressing tender feelings easily and being romantic.

Those with the highest levels of self-esteem characterized themselves as forceful, self-sufficient, outgoing, and ambitious. Approaching significance were express tender feelings easily, aggressive, and shy (negative correlation).

Most important for a lesbian's sense of self-worth were having close female

Table 6.31 Correlations among self-description variables and of these variables with self-esteem for males

Variable	Accomplished	Muscular	Compassionate	Outgoing	Aggressive	Express tender feelings	Forceful	Sexy looking	Affectionate	Competitive	Shy	Self-sufficient	Ambitious	Romantic	Athletic	Understanding	Movie star good looking	Self-esteem
Accomplished		.02	.26***	.10	.08	.09	.06	.02	.09	.08	−.08	.32***	.30***	.09	−.13	.02	−.05	.36***
Muscular			.04	.23***	.26***	.02	.22***	.54***	.02	.07	−.10	.15*	.15*	.03	.58***	.02	.42***	.06
Compassionate				.20**	.18**	.50***	.01	.16*	.57***	.10	.13	.20**	.31***	.55***	−.03	.44***	.04	.17**
Outgoing					.58***	.30***	.52***	.29***	.34***	.33***	−.35***	.25***	.38***	.27***	.18**	.19**	.25***	.27***
Aggressive						.21**	.64***	.28***	.26***	.36***	−.27***	.30***	.40***	.31***	.17**	.03	.25***	.28***
Express tender feelings							.15*	.21*	.68***	.09	−.10	.06	.20**	.54***	−.09	.26***	.10	.17*
Forceful								.22***	.11	.42***	−.29***	.25***	.37***	.19**	.14*	−.05	.17**	.27***
Sexy looking									.22**	.13	−.22**	.18**	.22**	.20**	.39***	.07	.64***	.17**
Affectionate										.18**	−.22**	−.00	.27***	.65***	.01	.29***	.12	.15*
Competitive											−.01	.13	.40***	.19**	.23***	−.11	.16*	.09
Shy												−.03	−.12	.02	−.03	.18**	−.22**	−.29***
Self-sufficient													.38***	.19**	.13	.11	.14*	.33***
Ambitious														.39***	.38***	.16*	.24***	.09
Romantic															−.00	.21**	.16*	−.00
Athletic																.03	.38***	.09
Understanding																	.00	−.00
Movie star good looks																		.15*
M	4.07	5.24	2.74	3.58	4.67	3.66	4.96	4.40	2.81	3.97	5.33	3.40	3.06	2.92	5.48	2.92	6.00	22.00
N	206	213	210	213	210	213	211	206	212	212	213	210	212	211	213	213	208	212

*p < .05. **p < .01. ***p < .001.

The most important components of self-worth among the males were having close male friends, a career, and academic success; the least, religion and having children. The former combine male friendships and success dimensions, whereas the latter are typically portrayed as feminine factors.

In Table 6.32 the correlations among the 12 self-worth variables and of those variables with self-esteem are presented. The highest correlations among the variables were between career and academic success and frequency of sex and good looks.

Those with the highest levels of self-esteem reported that most important for their sense of self-worth were a career, an active social life, and close male friends.

Predicting Male Self-Esteem

Five factors emerged from the self-descriptions factor analysis; their loadings are summarized in Table 6.33. The factors and their component parts were as follows: Shy, consisting of the shy variable; Muscular/Sexy, comprising the muscular build, sexy looking, movie star good looking, and athletic variables; Affectionate, comprising the affectionate, express tender feelings, romantic, and compassionate variables; Competitive, which included the competitive, forceful, and aggressive variables; and Accomplished, which included the accomplished and self-sufficient variables. These five factors significantly predicted gay self-esteem (Table 6.34). Two factors were major contributors: Accomplished and Shy (negative correlation).

The self-worth variables formed four factors (see Table 6.35): Friends, including the female friends and male friends variables; Religion, constituting the religion variable; Career/Academic, comprising the career and academic success variables; and Material Items, comprising the possessions, good looks, and sex frequency variables. These factors accounted for a significant portion of the self-esteem variation among the gay males (Table 6.36). In particular, the Career/Academic factor was a significant contributor; Material Items approached significance in a negative fashion.

Descriptive Results for Females

Lesbian youths were most likely to characterize themselves as affectionate, understanding, compassionate, and romantic, and least likely to characterize themselves as movie star good looking, shy, forceful, and having a muscular build. As with males, the "feminine" self-descriptors predominated over the more "masculine" terms.

Correlations among the 17 adjectives and of those adjectives with self-esteem are presented in Table 6.37. Several of the correlations were in excess of .70: muscular build with athletic, compassionate with affectionate, and sexy looking with movie star good looking.

Those with the highest levels of self-esteem characterized themselves as forceful, self-sufficient, outgoing, and ambitious. Approaching significance were express tender feelings easily, aggressive, and shy (negative correlation).

Most important for a lesbian's sense of self-worth were having close female

Table 6.32 Correlations among self-worth variables and of these variables with self-esteem for males

Variable	Career	Love relationship	Children	Social life	Frequent sex	Female friends	Physical looks	Academic success	Male friends	Relationship with parents	Religion	Possessions	Self-esteem
Career		.33***	.07	.30***	.19**	.11	.23***	.52***	.17**	.18**	.04	.26***	.22***
Love relationship			.14*	.23***	.30***	.08	.18**	.16*	.21**	.08	.05	.14*	.04
Children				.24***	.15*	.23***	.06	.08	.15*	.18**	.20**	.05	.04
Social life					.37***	.36***	.33***	.24***	.33***	.09	.18**	.33***	.14*
Frequent sex						.12	.47***	.21**	.21**	.11	-.02	.38***	-.04
Female friends							.14*	-.00	.30***	.18**	.08	.09	-.00
Physical looks								.19**	.28***	.13	.12	.41***	-.08
Academic success									.16*	.12	.08	.31***	.14
Male friends										.28***	.17**	.08	.02
Relationship with parents											.19**	.06	.05
Religion												.16*	.05
Possessions													.03
M	2.66	3.04	5.86	3.09	4.86	3.22	3.00	2.91	2.45	3.27	5.97	4.35	22.00
N	213	213	214	214	214	212	213	213	212	211	213	213	212

*p < .05.   **p < .01.   ***p < .001.

Table 6.33 Factor solution for self-description variables: Males

Factor	Shy	Muscular Sexy	Affectionate	Competitive	Accomplished
Shy	—	−.16	.03	−.27	−.02
Muscular Sexy		—	.15	.33	.12
Affectionate			—	.30	.27
Competitive				—	.28
Accomplished					—

Variable	Rotated factor pattern[a]				
Accomplished	−.16	−.14	.01	−.21	.83
Muscular	.04	.84	−.10	−.00	.02
Compassionate	.27	.04	.70	−.10	.28
Outgoing	−.32	.08	.24	.47	.09
Aggressive	−.21	.03	.09	.67	.11
Express tender feelings	−.19	−.04	.88	−.07	−.12
Forceful	−.26	.04	−.03	.74	.01
Sexy looking	−.20	.80	.18	−.14	.07
Affectionate	−.02	−.02	.91	.05	−.16
Competitive	.29	−.05	−.06	.90	−.17
Shy	.86	−.06	−.04	.06	−.06
Self-sufficient	.11	.13	−.20	.17	.75
Ambitious	.14	.06	.12	.50	.39
Romantic	.09	−.02	.74	.17	−.04
Athletic	.30	.77	−.21	.22	−.14
Understanding	.44	.15	.45	−.17	.23
Movie star good looks	−.17	.78	.08	−.11	−.04
Eigenvalue	1.41	2.31	2.62	1.87	1.46

[a]Standard regression coefficients.

Table 6.34 Regression predicting male self-esteem from self-description factors

Source	Full model				
	df	M^2	F	p	r^2
Model	5	244.93	13.61	.0001	.27
Error	185	17.99			

Factor	Parameter estimates			
	df	SE	t	p
Shy	1	.32	−3.53	.0005
Muscular Sexy	1	.33	.72	.47
Affectionate	1	.33	1.74	.08
Competitive	1	.36	.09	.93
Accomplished	1	.33	5.95	.0001

Table 6.35 Factor solution for self-worth variables: Males

Factor	Friends	Religion	Career/Academic	Material Items
Friends	—	.22	.30	.34
Religion		—	.14	.11
Career/Academic			—	.39
Material Items				—

Variable	Rotated factor pattern[a]			
Career	.05	−.09	.86	−.03
Love relationship	.36	−.19	.36	.09
Children	.50	.35	−.09	−.05
Social life	.43	−.05	.08	.42
Frequent sex	.14	−.13	−.01	.74
Female friends	.84	−.12	−.18	−.04
Physical looks	.03	.07	−.05	.76
Academic success	−.21	.04	.85	.05
Male friends	.55	.09	.18	−.02
Relationship with parents	.23	.50	.35	−.30
Religion	−.09	.86	−.08	.11
Possessions	−.22	.20	.08	.78
Eigenvalue	1.44	1.18	1.46	1.61

[a]Standard regression coefficients.

friends, a career, academic success, a lover relationship, and relationship with parents. Relatively unimportant were religion, having children, and material possessions.

Table 6.38 presents the correlations among the self-worth variables and of those variables with self-esteem. The self-worth variables most closely related included being in a lover relationship with frequency of sex and an active social life with good looks.

Table 6.36 Regression predicting male self-esteem from self-worth factors

	Full model				
Source	df	M^2	F	p	r^2
Model	4	82.36	3.38	.01	.06
Error	197	24.34			

	Parameter estimates			
Factor	df	SE	t	p
Friends	1	.38	.66	.51
Religion	1	.36	.63	.53
Career/Academic	1	.39	3.26	.001
Material Items	1	.39	−1.59	.11

Table 6.37 Correlations among self-description variables and of these variables with self-esteem for females

Variable	Accomplished	Muscular	Compassionate	Outgoing	Aggressive	Express tender feelings	Forceful	Sexy looking	Affectionate	Competitive	Shy	Self-sufficient	Ambitious	Romantic	Athletic	Understanding	Movie star good looking	Self-esteem
Accomplished		.02	.28**	.12	.01	.18	.14	.07	.13	.18	.03	.16	.28**	.15	-.04	.16	.08	.10
Muscular			.11	.26**	.32***	.00	.01	.48***	.15	.22*	.07	.35***	.29**	.18	.78***	.11	.25**	.13
Compassionate				.47***	.22*	.66***	.20*	.31**	.72***	.23*	-.03	.36***	.43***	.60***	.20*	.56***	.11	.11
Outgoing					.56***	.47***	.34***	.27**	.51***	.25*	-.38***	.35***	.39***	.47***	.23*	.46***	.13	.25**
Aggressive						.18	.53***	.18	.27**	.55***	-.29**	.27**	.34***	.39***	.44***	.22*	-.02	.19
Express tender feelings							.26**	.21*	.65***	.17	-.20*	.29**	.35***	.45***	.11	.47***	.12	.19
Forceful								.14	.16	.45***	-.26**	.17	.21*	.13	.16	.11	.10	.36***
Sexy looking									.28**	.16	-.01	.16	.35***	.23*	.38**	.28**	.70***	.10
Affectionate										.25**	-.17	.27**	.37***	.57***	.25**	.42***	.07	-.01
Competitive											-.07	.24*	.41***	.29**	.42***	.15	.07	.07
Shy												-.10	-.12	-.11	.10	-.08	.07	.19
Self-sufficient													.49***	.22*	.38***	.51***	-.07	.29**
Ambitious														.45***	.36***	.51***	.13	.23*
Romantic															.26**	.38***	.02	.10
Athletic																.21*	.21*	.08
Understanding																	-.03	.11
Movie star good looks																		.15
M	4.43	4.76	2.57	3.50	4.24	3.40	4.83	4.65	2.53	4.20	5.23	3.17	3.06	2.86	4.17	2.54	6.06	22.30
N	96	102	102	102	103	103	103	100	103	103	103	103	103	101	103	103	100	101

*p < .05. **p < .01. ***p < .001.

Table 6.38 Correlations among self-worth variables and of these variables with self-esteem for females

Variable	Career	Love relationship	Children	Social life	Frequent sex	Female friends	Physical looks	Academic success	Male friends	Relationship with parents	Religion	Possessions	Self-esteem
Career		.18	.03	.27**	.11	.07	.21*	.45***	.24**	.00	.04	.18	.04
Love relationship			.17	.12	.50***	.12	.13	.19	-.06	.23*	-.03	.15	-.03
Children				.27**	.23*	.13	.02	.11	.30**	.26**	.32***	.19	.09
Social life					.44***	.27**	.46***	.30**	.14	.13	-.01	.20*	-.05
Frequent sex						.33***	.38***	.32***	.14	.17	-.10	.20*	.04
Female friends							.18	.14	.20*	.08	-.06	.06	.05
Physical looks								.37***	.09	.13	-.09	.40***	-.18
Academic success									.05	.13	.05	.15	-.10
Male friends										.29**	.31***	.07	.07
Relationship with parents											.25**	.34***	.20*
Religion												-.04	-.02
Possessions													.07
M	2.36	2.95	5.86	3.47	4.94	1.68	3.53	2.75	4.03	3.02	6.59	5.31	22.30
N	103	103	98	103	102	103	102	102	103	103	103	103	101

*p < .05.   **p < .01.   ***p < .001.

Only one variable, relationship with parents, was significantly correlated with self-esteem.

Predicting Female Self-Esteem

Five factors were retained from analysis of the self-descriptions variables (see Table 6.39). These were Muscular, comprising the muscular build, athletic, and self-sufficient variables; Competitive, comprising the accomplished, competitive, and forceful variables; Good Looking, comprising the movie star good looking and sexy-looking variables; Affectionate, comprising the compassionate, affectionate, express tender feelings, understanding of others, and romantic variables; and Shy, including the shy variable. The regression model predicting lesbian self-esteem was significant (Table 6.40). The only significant factor was Shy (negative correlation).

Table 6.41 presents the loadings for the five factors derived from the factor analysis of the self-worth variables. The factors and components were as follows: Female Friends, formed from the female friends variable; Religion, comprising the religion, children, and male friends variables; Relationships, formed from the

Table 6.39 Factor solution for self-description variables: Females

Factor	Muscular	Competitive	Good Looking	Affectionate	Shy
Muscular	—	.35	.20	.37	−.28
Competitive		—	.14	.43	−.36
Good Looking			—	.13	−.07
Affectionate				—	−.39
Shy					—

Variable	Rotated factor pattern[a]				
Accomplished	−.31	.82	.08	.13	.33
Muscular	.94	−.15	.15	−.11	.05
Compassionate	−.10	.07	.07	.93	.11
Outgoing	.17	−.03	.06	.41	−.50
Aggressive	.42	.26	−.13	−.11	−.55
Express tender feelings	−.25	−.02	.07	.85	−.12
Forceful	−.10	.58	.11	−.20	−.51
Sexy looking	.20	−.03	.80	.19	−.02
Affectionate	.04	−.11	.06	.86	−.03
Competitive	.22	.77	−.09	−.12	−.06
Shy	.19	.19	.00	−.01	.91
Self-sufficient	.56	.08	−.22	.34	.10
Ambitious	.30	.38	−.01	.36	.07
Romantic	.05	.04	−.10	.64	−.13
Athletic	.93	−.00	.02	−.04	.07
Understanding	.07	−.01	−.14	.80	.09
Movie star good looks	−.05	.05	.95	−.09	.01
Eigenvalue	2.11	1.41	1.62	2.79	1.45

[a]Standard regression coefficients.

Table 6.40 Regression predicting female self-esteem from self-description factors

	Full model				
Source	df	M^2	F	p	r^2
Model	5	53.34	3.36	.008	.17
Error	80	15.86			

	Parameter estimates			
Factor	df	SE	t	p
Muscular	1	.49	.24	.81
Competitive	1	.51	1.30	.20
Good Looking	1	.44	.63	.53
Affectionate	1	.54	−.96	.34
Shy	1	−.48	−3.16	.002

relationships and sex frequency variables; Career/Academic, formed from the career and academic success variables; and Material Items, formed from the possessions and good looks variables. These five factors did not contribute a significant portion of the lesbian self-esteem level (Table 6.42).

Table 6.41 Factor solution for self-worth variables: Females

Factor	Female Friends	Religion	Relationships	Career/ Academic	Material Items
Female Friends	—	.08	.32	.21	.30
Religion		—	.06	.05	.13
Relationships			—	.25	.35
Career/Academic				—	.24
Material Items					—

Variable	Rotated factor pattern[a]				
Career	.03	.02	−.09	.91	−.04
Love relationship	−.11	.04	.91	.06	−.07
Children	.21	.62	.27	−.15	.01
Social life	.53	−.15	.09	.03	.31
Frequent sex	.38	−.08	.68	−.09	.04
Female friends	.83	.02	−.00	−.05	−.15
Physical looks	.26	−.26	−.11	.11	.72
Academic success	−.12	−.03	.33	.66	.06
Male friends	.46	.62	−.37	.21	−.02
Relationship with parents	−.21	.49	.17	−.05	.55
Religion	−.19	.78	−.02	.02	−.08
Possessions	−.15	.05	−.04	−.06	.89
Eigenvalue	1.32	1.70	1.35	1.23	1.41

[a]Standard regression coefficients.

Table 6.42 Regression predicting female self-esteem from self-worth factors

Source	df	M^2	F	p	r^2
		Full model			
Model	5	8.85	.45	.81	.03
Error	87	19.74			

Factor	df	SE	t	p
		Parameter estimates		
Female Friends	1	.50	.26	.80
Religion	1	.46	1.32	.19
Relationships	1	.51	− .18	.86
Career/Academic	1	.49	.45	.66
Material Items	1	.52	.14	.89

DISCUSSION

Sociodemographic Characteristics

Overall, the assessed sociodemographic variables had relatively little influence on the self-esteem level of the lesbian and gay youths sampled. The correlations of these enduring characteristics were slightly stronger for the lesbians than the gay males and for specific categories (e.g., hometown community).

Although age is a frequently cited variable in studies with gay men and lesbians, few studies have explored the influence of age on self-esteem level during the years of adolescence and youth. During the adult years, self-esteem apparently increases slightly for gay males with advancing age. In the current sample, from middle adolescence to the young adult years no age trends were apparent for the youths. Although few others have so reported, the most influential sociodemographic factor with the current sample would appear to be educational status. Independent of age, high levels of educational achievement were associated with positive self-esteem. Perhaps this is due to the youthful age of the population, a time when education is central to the lives of the individuals, or to the fact that many of the youths were currently enrolled in college at data collection time.

The reports of Weinberg and Williams (1974) and Ferguson and Finkler (1978) with adults generally were not supported with the current data. Gay and lesbian youths from prestigious-occupation families did not have higher self-esteem than others. This may be due to the fact that for the adults in the Weinberg and Williams study social status was an achieved marker, whereas for the present youths social status was an ascribed characteristic, bestowed by the family and thus not consequential for feelings about the self (Demo & Savin-Williams, 1983).

In most respects, knowledge of these sociodemographic characteristics added little to understanding the self-esteem of gay and lesbian youths. Only educational level attained appeared influential, approaching significance for both sexes. Apparently, one must turn more inward from these sociologically based factors to characteristics of the individual.

Attitudes and Interests

The assessed attitudes and interests were poor predictors of self-esteem level. With one exception, none was significantly correlated with self-esteem scores. That exception was political liberalism among the males.

Perhaps not surprisingly, given the current climate of liberal and conservative attitudes toward homosexuality, gay males who reported a liberal political philosophy had the highest level of self-esteem. To claim that one is conservative and gay is in direct opposition to the widespread finding (see review in Herek, 1984) that those least accepting of homosexuality tend to be politically, sexually, and religiously conservative. Thus, given these seemingly incompatible components, of being a gay conservative, it is not surprising that those most conservative have difficulty accepting a positive view of the self. This relationship was not, however, characteristic of the females. I do not have a plausible explanation except to suggest that perhaps the tie between the political and the personal are not as intertwined for females as they are for males. Certainly, the relationship between political ideology and self-evaluation would appear to be a useful area for future research.

Yet, political ideology is an infrequently assessed correlate of self-evaluation in previous studies of gay men and women. In fact, I could not find another study that related the two attitudes. The measure used in this study was a very general continuum spanning the range of liberal to conservative; a more specific political question relating to feminism produced few group differences among youths of either sex in predicting self-esteem level.

Results from the present study support the findings of Weinberg and Williams (1974): Religiosity and level of self-acceptance are relatively independent of each other. Interest in and skilled at athletic activities had little relationship to self-esteem levels among gay males, but among lesbians the correlation between the two was the highest for any of the variables (but still not significant). This difference will be explored further in Chapter 9.

Gay-Related Activities and Attitudes

Congruent with previous research on gay men (Hammersmith & Weinberg, 1973; Harry & DeVall, 1978; Miller, 1978; Weinberg, 1983; Weinberg & Williams, 1974), the male youths in this study who did not want to give up their homosexuality, even if they had the opportunity to do so, had the highest level of self-esteem. In combination with active participation in gay rights and activities, an Activism factor emerged that approached significance in predicting self-esteem scores among the gay males in the sample. Thus, positive attitudes toward oneself and one's sexual orientation and outward confirmation of that sexual orientation were associated with each other. Consistent with findings for political liberalism, these relationships were not characteristic of the lesbian youths. As will be more apparent below, the basis for a lesbian's self-evaluation resides with other issues.

Dank (1973) warned readers not to push a young male adolescent to make sense of his either explicit or subconscious sexual attractions to members of the same sex. At this age he is particularly sensitive to negative terms used by peers, such as "fag" and "sissy," that serve to insult and ridicule. Thus, he is likely to refrain from putting himself in that category in order to preserve his sense of self-worth.

On the other hand, the research of Harry and DeVall (1978) concluded that those who defined themselves as gay at an early age had the highest level of self-esteem. Neither position was supported by the gay males in the current sample; self-definition as gay at an early age was statistically unrelated to self-esteem. Among the lesbians, however, one of the best predictors of self-esteem was an early recognition of homosexual attractions. These findings, combined with the fact that the male youths questioned in the present study, as well as in many other studies, tend to recognize homosexual feelings much earlier than females, suggest that the relatively few women who know they are lesbian at an early age are indeed a special group: long-time, self-recognized lesbians with high self-esteem.

Such lesbians may have positive self-evaluations because they are more insightful and thus more accepting of themselves and their personality development in general. Or, it might be argued, integrating sexual identity at a relatively early developmental time allows women a longer time period to come to terms with this difficult recognition. By late adolescence their psychological and social resources and support services (e.g., a lover relationship or the lesbian community) have developed to complement the psychological benefits of mental and emotional maturity that come with age and with living in a relatively positive climate for homosexuality (e.g., out of the home and in college).

The fact that these relationships were not corroborated by males is not easily interpretable. Perhaps a recognition and awareness of "deviant" sexual feelings during pre- and early adolescence is too early developmentally; that is, the young male's psychological skills and maturity may not be sufficiently developed to counter Dank's (1973) warnings concerning negative reactions of self and others to one's "deviance." Or perhaps males who recognized quite early their homosexuality were forced into awareness by others because of their gender-atypical behaviors and mannerisms. The relationships among homosexuality, high effeminacy, and low self-regard were reviewed in Chapter 2. Females, on the other hand, are "allowed" a greater degree of cross-gender activities and interests during childhood and early adolescence (a volleyball example is given in Savin-Williams, 1987a).

The relationship between degree of sexual orientation and self-esteem is extremely mixed in the empirical literature, with support for negative, positive, and no correlation. The lesbians showed no correlation: Those with some heterosexual interests had neither higher nor lower self-esteem than lesbians who were exclusively homosexual. Male youths, on the other hand, who claimed to be exclusively gay had the highest level of self-evaluation. These findings are understandable if one accepts the speculations that many gay males who express heterosexual interests do not yet feel comfortable with or have not yet accepted their homosexuality, thus reflecting self-doubt and self-denigration and that females are more naturally bisexual and thus those who report heterosexual interests are reflecting their flexibility in matters of sexual behavior and interest.

Congruent with the findings of other investigators (Harry & DeVall, 1978; Weis & Dain, 1979), there was little relationship between the number of sex partners, either same- or other-sex, and self-esteem among the lesbian and gay youths. Thus, neither the stereotype that gay men and lesbians are promiscuous because they have low self-esteem nor the stereotype that those who avoid sex do so because of low self-evaluation was supported by the data. Apparently, factors other than self-esteem (e.g., sex drive, moral values, opportunities, and personality characteristics) determine the number of heterosexual and homosexual sexual relations that youths have.

There was also little apparent connection between self-evaluation and many of the gay-related political and social activities assessed by the GAL Q. These "no findings" are important given the dearth of research data on these issues, regardless of the age of the population.

Support of Family and Friends

Gay youths with the highest levels of self-esteem felt accepted by their mother, male and female friends, and their academic advisor; they also believed they had a large number of heterosexual friends. The first and last relationships barely reached acceptable levels of significance. In these matters the data are consistent with aspects of the literature cited in Chapter 5. Despite these correlations, the support variables did not account for a significant percentage of the variation in self-esteem among the male youths. The study results suggest that having straight friends and feeling acceptance from them, although associated with positive feelings about oneself, are not sufficient factors to predict high self-esteem. The nonsignificant regression analysis may reflect the fact that a third factor (e.g., a reporting style or another personality variable) accounts for the significant correlations between self-esteem and support variables. The nonsignificant relationships between self-evaluation and acceptance from gay, lesbian, and bisexual friends and between self-evaluation and number of gay, lesbian, and bisexual friends are counter to the theoretical perspectives of Weinberg and Coleman.

Data from the lesbian sample are also not particularly congruent with either Weinberg's sociological or Coleman's psychological perspective. On the other hand, the support variables did predict lesbian self-esteem level. Those who viewed themselves in a positive fashion had many bisexual but few gay friends. Having many bisexual friends of both sexes was a significant predictor of positive self-esteem. Perhaps having bisexual friends, which was an unusual occurrence for both the lesbian and gay youths, represents an extraordinary achievement. A sense of a secure self may allow one to befriend those who may be most threatening—those with ties to both the gay and straight worlds—and to maintain learning opportunities by crossing both worlds. Lesbian youths with high self-esteem may find this less troublesome. The near significance of an accepting family for positive self-esteem appears more intuitively and theoretically sensible. Even though the results reported in Chapter 8 document the importance of the family in terms of coming out and feeling comfortable with one's sexual orientation, the results are weak in terms of a lesbian's self-esteem.

Love and Love Affairs

There was a striking difference between the lesbian and gay youths in the importance of love affairs for self-evaluation. The self-esteem of the lesbians was essentially unrelated to any of the relationship variables. Those in a current love affair and those who maintain long relationships tended to have slightly higher self-esteem levels.

In contrast, self-esteem among the gay youths was significantly predicted by the love affair factors. Most important were a large number of love affairs, including a current one, and a high percentage of homosexual rather than heterosexual love affairs, including the first affair. Unrelated to positive self-esteem were the longevity of affairs and starting early in life with a love affair.

The male youths thus confirm a common finding in the literature, that those in a relationship have more positive views of the self. However, the issue is more complex than whether one is in or out of a relationship. Equally important is that love relationships have been primarily with other males and not females and that one has had many relationships, from an early age. Counter to the literature (Dickey, 1961; Weinberg & Williams, 1974; Wilkins, 1981), however, long-lasting relationships did not predict positive self-evaluation. Thus, rather than being singularly coupled, as Silverstein (1981) suggested is healthy for adult gays, gay youths appeared to feel more "chosen" if they were chosen early and frequently. The nature of the causal pathway—whether relationships enhance self-esteem or whether those with a positive view of the self are more likely to pursue other men—remains unaddressed by this research. For example, either or both of two statements are plausible: (a) Low self-esteem leads male youths to pursue heterosexual relationships, perhaps because by such endeavors their homosexuality is denied and they can claim to be "normal," and (b) engaging in heterosexual relationships enhances failure experiences and feelings of being untrue to one's natural inclinations, thus reinforcing a negative self-image.

The empirical literature regarding these issues among lesbians is nearly nonexistent. Given the importance of relationships to women (see Chapter 9), it is somewhat surprising to discover the relative independence of self-esteem and the love affairs variables. During adolescence other relationships besides romantic ones (e.g., friendships and family support) are important for self-evaluation as a good or bad person. These issues are prime candidates for more in-depth investigations than the current one was able to provide.

Self-Descriptions and Self-Worth

Both lesbians and gay males in the sample describe themselves in terms conventionally thought of by American society as feminine: romantic, affectionate, compassionate, and understanding of others. Least attributed to the self were shyness, movie star good looking, muscular build, athleticism (males), and forcefulness (females); all but the first are typical masculine characteristics. Thus, in their self-reports the lesbian youths did not confirm Ponse's (1980) view that lesbians possess a high level of qualities such as competence, assertiveness, and aggressiveness traditionally defined as masculine. The gay males described themselves as cultural stereotypes would assume, in a feminine fashion. But counter to these stereotypes, good looks and muscular build were seldom noted as frequent descriptors. As a group, the youths clearly saw themselves as warm, affectionate individuals with a concern for others; they deemphasized their physical attractiveness and assertiveness. The self-characterizations presented by these youths certainly would make them prime candidates as best friends, if not good lovers.

On the other hand, and quite strikingly, the best predictors of elevated levels of self-esteem for both gay males and lesbians were not the "feminine" characteristics that they frequently attributed to the self but the "masculine" attributes: ambitious, aggressive, forceful, outgoing, self-sufficient, accomplished (males), and sexy looking (males). Shyness was negatively related to self-esteem. There were a few exceptions, expressing tender feelings easily and being compassionate (males), but generally the youths in the sample viewed self-esteem and masculine attributes as emanating from the same "underlying construct."

This finding substantiates the view held by social scientists aware of sex bias in research that self-esteem is a masculine construction. To have extremely high levels of self-esteem would appear to be discrepant with how these gay youths view themselves. Yet, the self-esteem level of the lesbians (22.3) and gay males (22.0) is certainly not deficient when compared with the self-esteem scores of other samples of high school and college age youths, which usually range from 20 to 23 on the Rosenberg Self-Esteem Scale.

When asked to rate various aspects of self-worth for their centrality, academic and career success were important for both the female and male youths. These instrumental components were complemented by expressive, interpersonal elements, especially among the lesbians: close female friends and relationships with parents and a lover. Same-sex friendships were critical for the gay males as well. Unimportant were the more traditional, perhaps heterosexual, issues of religion, having children, and material possessions (females only).

These components of self-worth were relatively unimportant in predicting self-esteem among the lesbians. That is, differentiation among the lesbians on the self-worth variables was not related to their self-esteem level. Among the males the regression model was significant, primarily as a result of those who reported that academic and career successes were important for their sense of self-worth. But in neither case was a high percentage of the variance of self-esteem accounted for by the self-worth variables.

On the other hand, personality variables—the self-descriptors—accounted for far more of the self-esteem variance. Thus, to predict the self-esteem of both lesbian and gay youths, more important than their professed academic and career goals and their interpersonal relationships were personality characteristics that they attributed to the self. Perhaps this is not surprising if one assumes that self-esteem is, after all, a personality characteristic of a person, an enduring trait stable over time and settings. This fundamental issue of the stability of self-esteem and its status as a personality trait has been addressed in previous research (Savin-Williams & Demo, 1984).

Apparently, possessing high self-esteem was not considered a high priority, especially for the lesbians. Although the "masculine" self-worth components of academic and career success were important for the youths, they either did not predict self-esteem level (lesbians) or were relatively unimportant factors for self-esteem (gay males). Equally central for the youths were close, intimate personal relationships with friends, lovers, and parents. The gay and lesbian youths thus appeared to have bridged important human conditions. As a group they (a) maintained an adequate self-esteem level without becoming a slave to it; (b) saw themselves as warm, compassionate individuals who reject the attributions of aggression and physical attractiveness, thus countering heterosexual stereotypes of them; and (c) valued both personal and interpersonal success. Depending on one's philosophical and political leanings, these characteristics would appear to be optimally healthy for an individual's psychological health and for the health of society.

CONCLUSIONS

By way of summary, the modal gay and lesbian youths in the present sample are briefly described below, focusing on "average" responses given on the GAL Q. Although this presentation counters one of the major points that is pursued in Chapter 10, diversity, it serves as an overall characterization of the youths and a review of the major findings in this chapter.

Male

The average male youth in the sample was 20 years old with 14 years of education. Physically, he matured "on time." He grew up in a fairly well-to-do small town family. Oriented to neither religion nor sports, he was fairly liberal in political ideology.

He tended to be exclusively homosexual, felt that his sexual orientation was present at an early age, and believed his homosexuality was beyond his control to change, even if he wanted to (just under one-half of the males wished they could change to heterosexuality). The modal gay youth was relatively noninvolved in gay rights and gay/lesbian socialization activities, but he did go to a gay bar once a month. Up to this time in his life the modal youth had sex with 1 female and 6 to 10 males.

His friends were most likely to be other gay males and heterosexuals, in general, more males than females. The average male youth felt greatest acceptance from heterosexuals who were peer friends rather than parents. He had had either one or two love affairs in his first 20 years of life and he had a 50–50 chance of being in a current affair at the time of data collection. His first love relationship began around 17 years of age and lasted just under a year. Having a love relationship with a female sometime in his past would not have been unusual.

The average gay youth described himself as romantic, understanding of others, compassionate, affectionate, and ambitious. Relatively uncharacteristic were having movie-star good looks or being athletic, shy, or muscular. Most important for his sense of self-worth were having male friends and career/academic success. Of little importance were religion and having children.

The modal gay male was most likely to have high self-regard if he described himself as accomplished, self-sufficient, affectionate, romantic, and not shy; important to his sense of self-worth were career/academic success but not possessions, good looks, and frequency of sex. He was out to others, had had a large number of love affairs (including a current one), and had experienced a large percentage of his affairs (including his first) as homosexual.

Female

In terms of sociodemographics, the average lesbian youth was nearly identical to the average gay youth: a White, 20-year-old, with 14 years of education, pubertal onset at age 12 years, middle to upper middle class home, and reared in a small or middle-sized town. Compared with the typical male, the average lesbian was less religious, more liberal politically, more sports oriented, and more desirous of children.

The modal female youth recognized significant heterosexual interest, first felt her homosexuality during early adolescence, expressed little interest in giving up her sexual orientation, and was as likely as not to feel that she had control over her homosexuality. The average lesbian in the study was moderately active in gay rights, lesbian/gay organizations, and socialization with other lesbians and gays. She went to a lesbian bar two to three times per month. Sexual partners were equally split between males and females—two to three of each during her lifetime.

Her friendships were primarily with other females, both lesbian and straight. Acceptance was felt most strongly from friends and academic advisors, but not from parents.

The modal lesbian had a 50–50 chance of being in a current love affair, which was likely to be either her second or third love affair. Her first love affair began when she was 16.6 years of age and it was equally likely to be with a male as with a female. Her relationships lasted an average of 15 months.

The modal lesbian most frequently characterized herself as affectionate, understanding, compassionate, and romantic—but not as movie star good looking, shy, forceful, or muscular. For her sense of self-worth close female friends, academic/career success, lovers, and parents were most important; religion, children, and material possessions were least important.

Only two of the eight factor clusters distinguished the modal high self-esteem lesbian from her peers: Self-Description and Support of Family and Friends. She described herself as being not shy, having a large number of bisexual friends, and feeling accepted by family members.

7

Predicting Coming Out and Self-Esteem

OVERVIEW

In the broadest sense, self-disclosure refers to the act of sharing, both verbally and nonverbally, one's thoughts and feelings to another. These revelations may be of little or extreme importance; if the latter, then they may affect one's psychological well-being. In some cases the object of self-disclosure may be oneself. That is, an individual may recognize aspects of the self that heretofore have been neglected or perhaps actively suppressed. In the literature on homosexuality both coming out to self and coming out to others have been of theoretical and empirical interest. Although some writers have equated the two or have not adequately separated and considered the significance of each, developmental sequences that incorporate both dimensions have been constructed. These were reviewed in Chapter 3.

In this chapter, coming out is first presented as a multidimensional, behavioral construct. Then the relationships of a number of variables to coming out are explored, including sociodemographic characteristics, attitudes, activities, support, love affairs, and self-perceptions. Finally, the connecting link between coming out and self-esteem is made. Chapter 8 examines these issues more specifically in the context of coming out to one's parents.

COMING OUT AS MULTIDIMENSIONAL

Literature

A generalized, global measure of coming out is the usual assessment choice of researchers, although several have distinguished various dimensions based on the recipient's relationship to the gay person (e.g., family members, work or professional colleagues, peers, or employer). My concern here is in noting the relationships among those one claims one is out to, thus addressing the question, Is there a generalized "outness factor," or does it matter what the target's relationship is to the youth?

It is common to define coming out solely in behavioral terms, focusing on the object (to whom) or the number (to how many). Hooker (1965) was one of the first to define coming out in this manner—as a "debut," when an individual identifies the self publicly for the first time in the presence of other homosexuals. Plummer's (1975) definition of coming out stressed the decision to allow oneself to be identified as gay in the heterosexual world (which most models would place conceptually as a later developmental event than acknowledging oneself to other gays).

An important distinction was made by the sociologists Weinberg and Williams (1974) between "being known about" and "passing." Being known about refers to how many classes of others (e.g., family members, work associates, neighbors, and heterosexual friends) suspect or know an individual is homosexual as judged by a subjective assessment of the person. Bell and Weinberg (1978) used the measure as well to assess "overtness." More common is to consider passing, that is, whether the person has disclosed his or her sexual orientation to others (and to whom). Of critical importance is the issue of concealment: "I do not care who knows" or "From how many heterosexuals do you conceal your homosexuality?" (Weinberg & Williams, 1974). Whereas overtness refers to how many people know, passing considers the person's desire to reveal or not to reveal and thus is less of a number count.

Myrick (1974b) based self-disclosure scores on the sum of how many groups of individuals have been told. The range of revelation was from "lied to keep them from knowing" to full disclosure. In a second publication (Myrick, 1974a), the sample of men were grouped into four categories: covert–covert (no one knows and individual tries to conceal), overt–covert (no attempt to conceal, but no one knows), covert–overt (in general terms a few friends know), and overt–overt (all know).

Variations on these themes have emerged, focusing primarily on out-to-whom issues. Many have comparable checklists that include various categories (Elliot, 1982; Fitzpatrick, 1983; Hencken, 1985; McKirnan & Peterson, 1986; Nemeyer, 1980; O'Carolan, 1982), whereas others focus on specific categories, such as family members (Cramer, 1986; Grabert, 1985) or sexual partners (Braaten & Darling, 1965; Ferguson & Finkler, 1978). Ferguson and Finkler (1978) distinguished between personal outness, which they defined as involvement with another lesbian or telling just a few others, and overtness, which they defined as a public declaration such as joining a lesbian organization. Similarly, Lee (1977) noted stages of signification (self-label), coming out (disclosing to others), and going public. His focus was primarily on the last, which involved no concealment from others.

Hencken (1985) supported Weinberg's (1978) finding that frequently one first comes out behaviorally to a sexual partner. His data indicated that one tends to disclose first to same-sex and -orientation friends, especially intimate friends. Next, according to Hencken, are nuclear family, then business associates, then other relatives. There is much variability, however, in this order, depending on one's particular circumstances. Generally, one comes out to mother before to father (Grabert, 1985), perhaps because children tend to have more distant relationships with their father than with their mother (Fitzpatrick, 1983).

There is also general agreement that it is most difficult and yet most important in terms of identity development to come out to family members (Nemeyer, 1980). Cohen-Ross (1985) noted that for all identity groups coming out to mother, to other immediate family members, and to homosexual friends was the most important sequence. Thus, it is critical to distinguish among (a) who is told earliest, (b) who is most difficult to come out to, and (c) who is most important to tell. These three are likely to vary within and across individuals depending on one's developmental issues, what is most critical in one's life at a particular moment in time, and that person's characteristics, such as social class, religious values, and temperament.

In this section the primary focus is on addressing the unity of the behavioral component of coming out: Is there one general coming-out concept or does it vary in regard to the recipient of the self-disclosure? The literature, although not of one voice, generally supports a sequential pattern of disclosure. Issues of importance are addressed in Chapter 8.

Present Study Results

Males

Table 7.1 presents the correlations among items used to assess coming out (see Chapter 4). All correlations were significant at the .001 level. Clearly, if mother knew, father knew. Almost all gay males were out to their best heterosexual female and male friends; more were out to mother than father. In fact, father ranked next to last, just ahead of academic advisor/professor.

To assess the degree to which these measures of coming out were related to each other, factor analyses with oblique rotations were conducted. Among males, one factor emerged, Openness (see Table 7.2).

Females

Table 7.3 summarizes the correlations among the disclosure variables. Sixteen of the 21 coming-out correlations were significant; the highest was between mother knows and father knows. Academic advisor/professor was not significantly

Table 7.1 Correlations among coming-out variables for males

Variable	Mother	Father	Sibling	Male friend	Female friend	Professor	Open gay
Mother	—	.71*	.49*	.43*	.46*	.36*	.53*
Father		—	.48*	.44*	.43*	.36*	.48*
Sibling			—	.40*	.41*	.35*	.45*
Male friend				—	.60*	.39*	.51*
Female friend					—	.36*	.57*
Professor						—	.44*
Open gay							—
M	2.76	2.52	2.89	3.20	3.46	2.06	2.79
N	209	202	202	189	202	155	213

*p < .001.

Table 7.2 Correlations of coming-out variables with coming-out factors for gay males and lesbians

	Variable							
Factor	Mother	Father	Sibling	Male friend	Female friend	Advisor	Open gay	Eigen-value
Males								
Openness[a]	.81	.78	.70	.72	.75	.64	.82	3.92
Females								
General/Family Openness[a]	.63	.89	.81	.26	−.19	.28	.71	2.29
Open to Friends[a]	.21	−.15	−.05	.44	.88	.54	−.09	1.20

[a]Standard regression coefficients.

Table 7.3 Correlations among coming-out variables for females

Variable	Mother	Father	Sibling	Male friend	Female friend	Professor	Open gay
Mother	—	.48***	.47***	.41***	.31**	.18	.36***
Father		—	.44***	.30**	.09	.20	.35***
Sibling			—	.22*	.10	.17	.33***
Male friend				—	.34***	.35**	.36***
Female friend					—	.31**	.21*
Professor						—	.36***
Open gay							—
M	2.87	2.31	2.93	3.34	3.68	2.47	2.89
N	100	97	99	86	101	77	103

*p < .05.   **p < .01.   ***p < .001.

correlated with any of the family variables. Most female youths were out to best heterosexual female and male friends, and more were out to closest sibling than to either mother or father, and more were out to an academic advisor/professor than to their father. Overall, fathers appeared to be the last to know.

Among the lesbian youths two factors, General/Family Openness and Open to Friends, emerged (see Table 7.2). They were correlated with each other at the .31 level.

PREDICTING THOSE WHO COME OUT

Literature

The extent to which gay males and lesbians are overt concerning their sexual orientation is influenced by a number of factors, some characteristic of the individuals and others related to aspects of the environments in which they live (Harry & DeVall, 1978). The process is, of course, reciprocal in nature: As the coming-out process is experienced, perceptions of the self and of the external world may undergo gradual or radical transformation. Perhaps the safest position is to conclude that the acquisition of a sexual identity is accompanied by changes of behaviors and attitudes.

In this section of the chapter the focus is on changes of behavior: The extent to which the coming-out process is related to sociodemographic characteristics, attitudes, gay-related activities, support received from family and friends, love affairs, and self-perceptions. These have been only sporadically addressed by empirical investigations.

Sociodemographic Variables

Numerous investigators have examined the various factors that influence the age at which an individual comes out (e.g., Dank, 1971) or have focused on how the coming-out experience differs as a function of age (e.g., de Monteflores & Schultz, 1978). McDonald (1982) reviewed studies that cite the ages at which various milestone events in the coming-out process occur. As noted in Chapter 3, first awareness of same-sex attractions frequently coincides with the onset of puberty; disclosure to others is usually a much later event, possibly delayed until the individual is an adult. But there are considerable individual variations in the timing and sequence of first awareness and disclosure to others. In studies spanning a range of ages, older respondents are generally more out than younger ones, presumably because they have had a longer time period in which to come out (Brady, 1985; Myrick, 1974a; Straver, 1976). A counter finding is the research of McKirnan and Peterson (1986). The age range of their sample was 17 to 72 years, and with increasing age the distribution of the sample significantly shifted from "completely open" to "closeted." The mean age of the completely open group was 33 years; of the closeted group, 41 years. These findings may reflect the large-scale consensus that the milestone events are occurring at chronologically earlier ages during the last two decades (Dank, 1971; Kimmel, 1978; McDonald, 1982; Smith, 1983), a critical development because Cramer (1986) demonstrated that the amount of time one is out is a better predictor of self-esteem than age per se.

Despite the wealth of information that correlates age with the development of a gay or lesbian identity, few studies have examined adolescent experiences in coming out, either relative to other ages of the life course or within the period of adolescence, except retrospectively. Brady (1985) reported in his sample of gay men that those in the earliest stages of the coming-out process were "students," presumably the youngest individuals in his study. The average age of initial homosexual behavior in a sample of male youths (ages 15 to 21 years) was 13.3 years; public disclosure occurred some 3 years later at the average age of 16.5 years (Rector, 1982). In the Netherlands the comparable ages were 13 and 15 years for gay males (G. Sanders, 1980). If the population of lesbians or gay males studied included adolescents, they were seldom examined separately or in relation to older members of the sample. Because many come out as adolescents or as young adults, more attention needs to be directed at this population.

In terms of social class, self-disclosure was more prevalent among students from upper class than from working class backgrounds in a Netherlands sample ages 15 to 26 years (Straver, 1976). Similarly, gay men in the United States who were in the "professional" class were furthest along in the coming-out process (Brady, 1985). Myrick's (1974a) data were in basic agreement: Covert–covert men were in the lowest occupational status categories. Unclear, however, is whether social class is independent of age; that is, those who are older may be more likely to have advanced in their career than younger individuals. Again, a counter finding was reported by McKirnan and Peterson (1986): Those in the higher categories of income and occupation were most closeted. Occupational status was unrelated to whether one was out to those most interpersonally close (friends and family) but strongly related to whether one was out to casual friends, co-workers, and acquaintances. They felt this was due to the pressures of homophobia in higher status occupations.

Ferguson and Finkler (1978) suggested that lower class lesbians most overt in their sexual orientation experience more anxiety than those who are not out. This relationship was not considered to be characteristic of higher social status lesbians. Studies that examine the socioeconomic background of the lesbian or gay youth's family in terms of its impact on the coming-out process are nonexistent.

Finally, it has been suggested that gay men and lesbians adapt most easily in the city, where anonymity protects them from social rejection, role models are more available, and heterogeneity and differentiation encourage a supportive milieu (Bell & Weinberg, 1978; Weinberg & Williams, 1974). Rural gay men and lesbians, who live in small communities in which everyone knows and interacts with everyone else and in which knowledge of one's purported deviancy, such as sexual orientation, spreads quickly throughout the community, may be less likely to openly disclose their identity to others (D'Augelli & Hart, 1987; Moses & Buckner, 1980). D'Augelli and Hart (1987) noted the problems in rural areas where gay and lesbian communities seldom exist, either for those just coming out or for people who have defined themselves as gay or lesbian for some time: "This invisibility is a result of justifiable fear and discomfort about others' reactions to disclosure of affectional orientation. Many rural gays fear discovery and possible rejection, worrying that any gay behavior will lead to exposure" (p. 82). Thus, it seems reasonable to assume that youth raised in the city would also be more willing to disclose their sexual orientation to others. Despite these assertions, researchers have generally not included issues of urban/rural rearing in their research designs on coming out.

Judging from the literature reviewed above, older youth and those reared in an urban environment should be most out. Social class data are conflicting as to their influence and little is known concerning the impact of two variables considered to be important during adolescence: educational level and pubertal onset date.

Attitudes and Interests

As noted in the self-esteem literature review, investigators seldom consider attitudes and interests as independent variables in their research. There are several exceptions in terms of coming out. With a sample of 102 Missouri lesbians, O'Carolan (1982) noted that the relationship between self-disclosure and feminism was not significant. With regard to religiosity, self-disclosure was highest when there was relatively little attachment to a church in a Netherlands sample (Straver, 1976). A single study explored the desire for children. Contrary to the hypothesized psychoanalytic prediction, Smith (1983) discovered in his sample of 117 gay males that there was no difference in motivation for wanting children; regardless of identity level, the majority of the sample wanted children.

Harry and DeVall (1978, p. 69) concluded, "The phenomenological event of self-definition seems to have stronger relationships with attitudes than does the behavioral event of coming out." Because the present study focused on the latter, I determined whether there were significant relationships between coming out and the variables in this category.

Gay-Related Activities and Attitudes

Several studies, with both lesbians (Elliot, 1982) and gay men (Cramer, 1986; McDonald, 1982), concluded that socialization within the gay and lesbian communities was more prevalent with increasing certainty of one's homosexuality. The best predictor of disclosure to others among a primarily Canadian lesbian population of 305 was political awareness and involvement (Elliot, 1982). Several writers have noted the particular importance of support within the lesbian community for a woman in the midst of her coming-out process (Ettorre, 1980; Ponse, 1980; Richardson, 1981b). The friendship ties are sources of romantic and sexual relationships, social norms for a lesbian identification, and lesbian role models. They enhance coming out as a positive experience. For both lesbians and gay men frequent bar patrons tended to be more out to others, except for those who went only to bars and not to other lesbian and gay activities (McKirnan & Peterson, 1987b).

Thus, recent evidence does not support an early position represented by Myrick (1974b). The overt homosexual men in his sample tended to be socially isolated from the gay subculture. Although they accepted their sexual orientation, by being publicly out the men had become isolated from both the larger social world and members of the gay community. Others may not be as overt and thus fear "guilt by association."

In terms of attitudes toward homosexuality, from a labeling perspective Weinberg (1983) maintained that coming to terms with one's sexual orientation is easier if one holds positive views toward that orientation. This is most likely to occur if one was reared in a tolerant atmosphere. But several investigations have not supported this view. Essentially the same attitudes toward homosexuality existed for both those who had and had not disclosed to parents, suggesting that holding positive attitudes toward homosexuality is not essential for disclosure to family members (Grabert, 1985). O'Carolan (1982) discovered that locus of control, the degree to which one feels in control of life's happenings and that it is oneself rather than fate that determines events, did not differentiate self-disclosure level among her Midwest sample of lesbians. Finally, Harry and DeVall (1978) reported that having negative attitudes toward homosexuality was not significantly related to either defining oneself as gay or coming out to others among gay men.

On the other hand, sharp differences have been noted between those who are out and those who are not. McDonald (1982, 1984) reported that males most identified as gay and out of the closet had the lowest levels of homophobic prejudice; those reticent to disclose to others felt guilt, anxiety, and shame about being homosexual. Similarly, Elliot (1982) found a positive correlation between certainty of lesbianism and good feelings concerning lesbianism in general. However, lesbians who recognized their homosexuality at an early age took a long time to establish a positive lesbian identity. In a study of clinical and nonclinical gay men and lesbians, those highest on self-disclosure were lowest on internalized fear of societal negative attitudes toward homosexuality and on distress over homosexual arousal and life-style. They were less likely than their closeted peers to desire heterosexual arousals or life-styles (Miranda, 1986).

One's placement on the homosexual–heterosexual continuum has been well documented in accounting for differences in overtness. Bell and Weinberg (1978) reported that those who rated themselves as exclusively homosexual were most willing to disclose their sexual identity to others. Compared with men who were less exclusively gay, they were less concerned with passing as heterosexual, less likely to engage in heterosexual behaviors and fantasies, and more known about (McDonald, 1982; Myrick, 1974b; Weinberg & Williams, 1974).

Among male youths, defining oneself as homosexual was related in Rector's (1982) dissertation study more to sexual behavior than it was to sexual feelings. There was a diversity of sexual feelings, including heterosexual ones, expressed by the youths, despite defining themselves as gay. The earlier a male defined himself as gay and came out to others the more likely he was to have engaged in teenage homosexual sex (Harry & DeVall, 1978). Gay men highest on self-disclosure had the most liberal attitudes toward sexual contacts outside of a relationship (Straver, 1976).

Thus, there is fairly strong support for the view that lesbians and gay males most involved in the lesbian and gay communities and who claim to be exclusively homosexual are most likely to be publicly out of the closet. Results on the relationship between self-disclosure and attitudes toward homosexuality are mixed, with studies supporting both a lack of consistent trends and a positive co-occurrence. Too few studies have examined number of sexual partners and age at which one first felt homosexual to suggest the relationship of these two variables with coming out.

Support From Family and Friends

Coming out may add a positive sense to the self-label lesbian or gay if one gains in the process support from family, co-workers, friends, and the lesbian and gay communities (Nungesser, 1983). In a sample of Netherlands gay men, those most out had positive relations with heterosexuals and an integrated friendship network of both straights and gays (Straver, 1976). From interviews with 20 male youths between 16 and 20 years of age (de Koning & Blom van Rens in Straver, 1976), it was found that neither the number of friends nor the amount of time spent socializing with them was as crucial as having people with whom problems could be discussed as one progressed through different phases of development. Aside from the literature cited in the preceding section and in Chapter 3, this assertion has seldom been tested. An exception is the research of McKirnan and Peterson (1987b), who found that lesbians and gay men who were most out had many confidants, individuals one could talk to intimately and turn to for help.

Love Affairs

Both the self-definitional and behavioral coming-out dimensions were significantly correlated with "experienced gay crushes" and "interests in other males during adolescence" in Harry and DeVall's (1978) study of gay men. In addition, defining oneself as gay at an early age was significantly and positively correlated with desire for establishing a long-term romantic relationship with another male and negatively correlated with heterosexual dating, crushes, and interests. In terms of actually having a relationship and coming-out status, the research of McKirnan and Peterson stands alone. They found no relationship between coupledness and outness among their 739 lesbians; among their 2,625 gay men there was a slight (statistically significant but of a low order) tendency for those most out to be in a romantic relationship (P. Peterson, personal communication, 1988).

Self-Descriptions

Relatively few studies of coming out have investigated issues of self-assessment in personality characteristics. In general, self-disclosure appears positively related to Bem's notion of femininity for both gay and lesbian college students (Bender, Davis, Glover, & Stapp, 1976). With a sample of 36 adolescents between the ages of 15 and 21 years, Rector (1982) found little relationship between the development of homosexual feelings and behaviors and psychological androgyny.[1] A self-disclosing group of gay males ages 18 to 58 years were most likely to reveal aspects of themselves to their parents in other areas of their lives (Grabert, 1985).

Present Study Results for Males

Descriptive

Table 7.4 presents the correlations of all study variables with the Openness factor. Thirty-three of the 70 correlations were significant beyond the .05 level. In terms of sociodemographic and attitude variables, males most open tended to be of advanced age, highly educated, early maturing, and liberal and feminist in ideology. Nearly all of the gay activities were significantly correlated with openness: Those most out tended to be exclusively homosexual, had felt their sexual orientation at an early age, were actively involved in the gay rights movement (highest of the 70 correlations), frequently went to gay bars, socialized with other gays and lesbians, attended gay and lesbian activities, read gay periodicals, would not give up their homosexuality even if they could, and had many male sexual partners. Similarly, most of the support of family and friends variables were significantly related to the Openness factor: Those most out felt acceptance from their mother, father, sibling, closest heterosexual female and male friends, and academic professor or advisor. They reported having many gay and lesbian friends and few bisexual male friends (number of bisexual female and heterosexual male and female friends was unrelated). Gay males who had had many love affairs were most likely to be open concerning their sexual orientation; none of the other affair variables was significantly related to Openness. Males most out described themselves as accomplished, outgoing, and understanding of others' feelings, but not as compassionate, expressing tender feelings easily, or affectionate. Finally, in terms of what is most important for one's self-worth, those most out responded being in a love relationship and having close male friends. The other 10 items were not significantly related.

Regression Models

Six of the seven factor regression models were significant in predicting coming out (Table 7.5). The only exception was the love affairs model. In descending order of importance, gay males most out

1. Were involved in political and social organizations with other gays and lesbians, had numerous homosexual encounters, were regular bar patrons, and felt their homosexual feelings were from an early age and beyond their control;
2. Had family members and friends who accepted their sexual orientation and reported having many friends;
3. Described themselves as accomplished and self-sufficient, but not as either competitive–forceful or affectionate–compassionate;
4. Were older, well educated, early maturing, and from wealthy urban families;

[1]Rector (1982) found that as a group the gay youths were above average on androgyny, using the Bem Sex Role Inventory.

Table 7.4 Correlation of all variables with openness factor for males and females

Variables	Males		Females	
	r	p	r	p
Age	.27	.003	−.15	.268
Education	.25	.006	−.14	311
Ed-age	.14	.134	.14	.298
Pubertal onset	−.25	.006	.11	.409
Hometown community	.10	.256	.30	.020
Parental occupation status	.16	.085	.02	.862
Religiosity	−.10	.296	.00	.984
Political outlook	.35	.001	−.12	.380
Feminism	.27	.002	.05	.701
Number of children desired	−.14	.195	−.30	.050
Sports	−.08	.404	−.03	.841
Sexual orientation	.36	.001	.51	.001
Age first felt homosexual	−.28	.002	−.18	.190
Give up desire	−.44	.001	−.41	.002
Beyond control	.16	.080	.02	.888
Gay rights	.64	.001	.53	.001
Gay/lesbian bars	.39	.001	−.04	.770
Gay/lesbian socialization	.44	.001	.35	.007
Gay/lesbian activities	.60	.001	.45	.001
Periodicals	.38	.001	.31	.017
Sex partners				
Number males	.23	.013	−.39	.003
Number females	−.06	.500	.20	.128
Mother	.21	.022	.30	.023
Father	.29	.002	.42	.001
Sibling	.39	.001	.52	.001
Female friend	.56	.001	.05	.727
Male friend	.53	.001	.39	.003
Professor	.36	.001	.37	.005
Gay friend	.30	.002	.27	.050
Lesbian friend	.24	.012	.13	.371
Bisexual male friend	−.19	.052	.05	.757
Bisexual female friend	−.05	.590	−.04	.787
Heterosexual male friend	−.09	.339	−.14	.322
Heterosexual female friend	.01	.918	−.19	.172
Number of love affairs	.21	.021	−.02	.857
Current affair	.00	.965	−.00	.991
Longevity	.00	.976	.04	.777
Age of first affair	.19	.143	−.02	.873
Sex of first lover	−.01	.930	.44	.003
Percentage of gay affairs	.14	.143	.34	.012
Accomplished	.23	.012	−.06	.681
Muscular	−.01	.920	−.00	.989
Compassionate	−.36	.001	.13	.327
Outgoing	.23	.011	.07	.598
Aggressive	−.09	.325	−.08	.537
Express tender feelings	−.30	.001	.23	.077
Forceful	−.00	.988	.14	.281
Sexy looking	−.08	.361	−.05	.706
Affectionate	−.26	.004	.15	.246
Competitive	−.09	.343	.01	.948

Table 7.4 (Continued)

Variables	Males		Females	
	r	p	r	p
Shy	−.09	.312	−.05	.680
Self-sufficient	.15	.114	.11	.401
Ambitious	.08	.398	−.02	.863
Romantic	.16	.087	−.02	.902
Athletic	−.04	.631	−.07	.617
Understanding	.19	.034	.02	.864
Movie star good looking	−.15	.101	.05	.730
Career	.13	.171	−.25	.063
Love relationship	.18	.052	−.11	.431
Children	−.11	.234	−.24	.083
Social life	.01	.945	−.23	.079
Frequent sex	−.15	.111	−.11	.402
Female friends	.13	.150	−.20	.142
Physical looks	−.14	.117	−.06	.661
Academic success	−.00	.993	−.20	.136
Male friends	.20	.031	−.27	.042
Parents	.11	.240	.15	.262
Religion	−.08	.405	−.11	.402
Possessions	.01	.922	.01	.968
Self-esteem	.21	.022	−.02	.860

5. Reported that material things such as possessions and good looks were not important to their sense of self-worth but that friends, career, and academics were;

6. Were politically liberal and supportive of the feminist movement.

Present Study Results for Females

Descriptive

Of the 70 study variables, 18 were significantly correlated with the General/ Family Openness factor (Table 7.4).[2] Lesbian youths most out tended to grow up in urban areas, wanted few children, claimed to be exclusively homosexual, participated in gay rights activities (the highest correlation of any variable), socialized with other lesbians and gays, attended lesbian and gay activities, read lesbian-related materials, had little desire to give up their sexual orientation, and seldom had sexual relations with males. In terms of support from family and friends, those most out felt accepted by their mother, father, sibling, close heterosexual male (but not female) friend, and academic advisor, and reported having few heterosexual female friends. Having many gay friends was related to whether or not a lesbian was out to others. Lesbians whose first sexual encounter was with a female and whose ratio of female to male love affairs was decidedly slanted toward females were most likely to report being out to others. The only self-description or self-

[2]In the correlational and regression analyses, the General/Family Openness factor was selected because of its considerably greater eigenvalue than the Open to Friends factor.

Table 7.5 Regression models: Predicting coming out for gay males

Source	Full model					Parameter estimates			
	df	M^2	F	p	r^2	df	SE	t	p
				Sociodemographics					
Model	3	3.42	4.11	.009	.11				
Error	104	.83							
Factor									
Pubertal Onset						1	.10	−1.95	.05
Age/Education						1	.09	2.20	.03
Hometown Community/									
Socioeconomic Status						1	.10	1.92	.06
				Attitudes and interests					
Model	1	3.58	3.95	.05	.04				
Error	88	.91							
Factor									
Liberalism						1	.10	1.99	.05
				Gay-related activities					
Model	4	13.55	26.80	.0001	.50				
Error	106	.51							
Factor									
Heterosexual Acts						1	.08	.56	.58
Activism						1	.07	7.88	.0001
Always Gay						1	.08	2.31	.02
Gay Bar/Sex						1	.07	2.38	.02
				Support of family and friends					
Model	4	8.27	13.77	.0001	.40				
Error	83	.60							
Factor									
Straight/Gay Friends						1	.09	1.91	.06
Bisexual Friends						1	.09	−1.39	.17
Mother/Sibling Accept						1	.09	2.10	.04
Friends Accept						1	.09	5.15	.0001
				Love affairs					
Model	3	.86	1.08	.37	.05				
Error	56	.79							
Factor									
Affair Length						1	.11	.69	.50
Gay Affairs						1	.11	.36	.72
Affair Number						1	.11	1.53	.13
				Self-description					
Model	5	4.01	3.97	.003	.16				
Error	104	1.01							
Factor									
Shy						1	.10	1.66	.10
Muscular/Sexy						1	.09	.42	.67
Affectionate						1	.10	−3.03	.003
Competitive						1	.11	−2.16	.03
Accomplished						1	.10	2.28	.02

Table 7.5 (Continued)

Source	Full model					Parameter estimates			
	df	M^2	F	p	r^2	df	SE	t	p
			Self-worth						
Model	4	2.38	2.49	.05	.08				
Error	114	.96							
Factor									
Friends						1	.10	2.03	.05
Religion						1	.10	−1.45	.15
Career/Academic						1	.10	1.69	.09
Material Items						1	.10	−2.07	.04

worth item that was significantly correlated with Openness for the youths was male friends as important (negative correlation) for their sense of self-worth.

Regression Models

Of the seven factor models accounting for lesbian coming out, three were significant and a fourth approached significance (Table 7.6). In descending order of importance, those most out

1. Were actively involved in the gay rights movement and organizations, socialized with other lesbians and gays, had few sexual relations with males, and did not want to give up their sexual orientation;
2. Felt accepted by family members and reported having many gay and lesbian friends;
3. Experienced love affairs that were primarily homosexual and not heterosexual, including their first love affair;
4. Reported that female and male friends were not important for their sense of self-worth.

RELATIONSHIP BETWEEN COMING OUT AND SELF-ESTEEM

Literature

Coming out has the potential to affect many dimensions of an adolescent's life, including personal and social issues such as emotional and psychological well-being, self-concept, identity, and relations with family, friends, and work colleagues (Nemeyer, 1980). In this section the focus is on the relationship between disclosing one's sexual orientation and one dimension of self-concept, self-esteem.[3]

[3]Other aspects of openness and overtness—the number of heterosexual and homosexual partners one has had, the age at which one first felt attraction to members of the same sex, and the degree to which one's sexual orientation is exclusively homosexual or contains some elements of heterosexuality—are addressed in Chapter 6.

Table 7.6 Regression models: Predicting coming out for lesbians

| Source | \multicolumn{5}{c}{Full model} | \multicolumn{4}{c}{Parameter estimates} |
	df	M^2	F	p	r^2	df	SE	t	p
\multicolumn{10}{c}{Sociodemographics}
Model	3	.66	.63	.60	.04				
Error	50	1.04							
Factor									
Hometown Community/									
Socioeconomic Status						1	.13	− 1.00	.32
Age/Education						1	.13	− .05	.96
Pubertal Onset/Ed-Age						1	.15	.83	.40
\multicolumn{10}{c}{Attitudes and interests}
Model	2	1.48	1.41	.26	.07				
Error	37	1.05							
Factor									
Liberalism						1	.17	.54	.59
Number of children desired						1	.17	− 1.64	.11
\multicolumn{10}{c}{Gay-related activities}
Model	5	5.95	12.71	.0001	.57				
Error	48	.47							
Factor									
Lesbian Bar/Sex						1	.09	− .80	.43
Heterosexual Acts						1	.10	− 3.86	.0003
Recently Lesbian						1	.11	− 1.33	.19
Activism						1	.10	4.78	.0001
Give Up Desire						1	.09	− 3.37	.002
\multicolumn{10}{c}{Support of family and friends}
Model	4	5.95	9.91	.0001	.52				
Error	37	.60							
Factor									
Lesbian/Gay Friends						1	.12	2.16	.04
Bisexual Friends						1	.12	− .61	.55
Female Friend Accepts						1	.12	1.66	.11
Family Accepts						1	.12	5.78	.0001
\multicolumn{10}{c}{Love affairs}
Model	3	4.23	5.25	.004	.28				
Error	40	.81							
Factor									
Lesbian Affairs						1	.14	3.73	.0006
Affair Length						1	.15	1.45	.15
Affair Number						1	.14	− 1.21	.23
\multicolumn{10}{c}{Self-description}
Model	5	.10	.15	.98	.02				
Error	42	.65							
Factor									
Muscular						1	.14	.48	.63
Competitive						1	.15	.38	.71

Table 7.6 (Continued)

Source	Full model					Parameter estimates			
	df	M^2	F	p	r^2	df	SE	t	p
Self-description (*continued*)									
Factor (*continued*)									
Good Looking						1	.12	.32	.75
Affectionate						1	.15	.63	.54
Shy						1	.14	−.17	.86
Self-worth									
Model	5	1.71	1.78	.14	.16				
Error	47	.96							
Factor									
Friends						1	.16	−2.02	.05
Religion						1	.15	−.55	.59
Relationship						1	.16	.37	.71
Career/Academic						1	.16	−1.61	.11
Material Items						1	.15	1.33	.19

The clinical psychologist Malyon (1981) traced the process of coming out primarily through changes in self-concept. The new self-awareness of coming out may temporarily create anxiety, leading to feelings of self-contempt, before an individual rejects the social stereotype of homosexuals as lonely and depressed. With a direct increase in self-esteem the individual shares "the secret" with more and more persons. One's self-concept may be quite vulnerable at this point, needing the support of friends, family, and perhaps a therapist. Eventually, an integrated identity, intimacy, and fulfilling relationships signify self-acceptance and positive self-esteem.

For Weinberg and Williams (1974) it is not passing per se that leads to poor self-regard but the fear and anxiety of exposure and anticipated discrimination that result in psychological problems. This is somewhat similar to the "uncomfortableness being gay" attitude that is described in Chapter 8. Weinberg and Williams noted, "Compared with less known-about homosexuals, the more known about are not found to have greater psychological problems, as many would expect. Thus, being known about is not the 'end of the world,' as many homosexuals fear" (1974, p. 260). When asked whether they acted publicly in ways that indicated their socialization to common homosexual practices and their subjective assessment of whether others knew that they were gay, there were few differences in psychological well-being among those high, medium, or low on these dimensions. Similarly, when Harry and DeVall (1978) asked a sample of Detroit men to reflect on their adolescence, neither the age of coming out to others, a behavioral event, nor the phenomenological event of defining oneself as gay (an issue of identity) at a young age was significantly related to self-esteem level.

Coming out thus apparently has little negative impact on psychological well-being, and a number of studies have documented the positive association between coming out and self-esteem. In research focusing on college students who came to the university clinic for psychological services, covert gay men displayed more intrapsychic tensions, social–psychological problems, and social introversion than did overt gay students (Braaten & Darling, 1965). Covert gay men were defined as those in the beginning stages of homosexual self-recognition: They experienced homosexual impulses, fantasies, and dreams and had not yet engaged in many overt homosexual behaviors. Overt gay men, by contrast, had had many homosexual encounters. In another sample of young adults, from the Netherlands, there was a strong correlation between acceptance of one's homosexual feelings and self-esteem among 132 males and 81 females (G. Sanders, 1980). The association between "manifesting oneself as a homosexual," taken to be disclosure to others in general, and self-esteem was, however, considerably lower.

Self-esteem was a positive, but low-order, correlate of self-disclosure in a sample of 188 gay men and lesbians (Miranda, 1986). One respondent in Friend's (1980) study of 43 gay men between the ages of 32 and 76 years said, "Coming out is something everyone should go through, because if they can handle that, they can handle anything"(p. 242). The correlation between self-esteem and coming out was positive and significant.

A recent survey of 3,400 Chicago area gay men and lesbians (McKirnan & Peterson, 1986, 1987a, 1987b, 1987c), solicited through area newspapers, bars, businesses, community organizations, mailing lists, and special events, documented the close link between psychological well-being and disclosure. Respondents were asked if they were out to each of nine groups (e.g., close friends, parents, co-workers). Those most closeted had the highest levels of social conflict (experienced stress with being gay or lesbian in social settings, such as work), personal conflict ("within myself" conflict), alienation, depression, and negative self-esteem. The correlations of the last two with outness, although significant, were relatively small.

With a sample of 276 middle-class Texas bar patrons between the ages of 29 and 52 years, the overt gay man, defined in terms of disclosure to others, was higher on self-acceptance and power and higher on social isolation than his covert peer (Myrick, 1974a). Covert–coverts had the most concern with self-esteem, self-acceptance, and status. They were likely to feel the most socially isolated, powerless, normless, and personally incompetent.

Since these seminal works a number of dissertations, including research with lesbians, have addressed the tie between coming out and self-esteem. They are essentially of one voice: Coming out to the self is related to positive and not negative self-esteem, but the relationship between disclosure to others and positive self-regard is mixed. The findings among lesbians are fairly consistent. For example, Elliot (1982) found a positive correlation between self-esteem and feelings about being a lesbian in a sample of 305 adults; self-esteem was not, however, a significant predictor of disclosure to others. O'Carolan (1982) confirmed the positive correlation between self-esteem and feelings about being a lesbian with a sample of 102 lesbians using the Coopersmith Self-Esteem Inventory and a measure of self-affirmation as self-disclosure. In a qualitative study of 25 lesbian women, self-disclosure (including aspects of coming out to self and to others) was a "critical factor" influencing self-acceptance (Nemeyer, 1980).

Several dissertation studies of gay men agree: Those most out to self are the best adjusted psychologically (Benitez, 1983, sample of 178 males). Psychological well-being (happiness, psychological health, sexual satisfaction, etc.) was found to correspond to movement beyond the initial tolerance stage of coming out to the later stages of acceptance, pride, and synthesis (Brady, 1985, sample of 225 men).

In a study of 215 gay men, McDonald (1984) reported that those most identified as gay and out of the closet had the optimal level of identity congruency. He concluded that the best adjusted men integrated and managed their personal identity, a process which entailed being "totally homosexual." It is unclear, however, whether self-esteem was higher as a result. More complex are the findings of Cramer (1986) with a sample of 93 gay males. The mean level of self-esteem was significantly higher for those who had disclosed to parents than for those closeted and not wanting out; the difference in self-esteem was not significant for those who were closeted and wanted out and the disclosers. Thus, congruent with the other dissertation research, Cramer's findings suggest that the primary issue is more related to self disclosure than other disclosure. However, he also reported that the longer one had been out to others the higher the self-esteem level. Generally, the literature appears fairly consistent in regard to the positive and intimate relationship between self-esteem and coming out to self. Less clear is the relationship between disclosure to others and self-esteem, especially among lesbians.

Present Study Results

Among males self-esteem was significantly correlated with general openness ($.27, p < .001$), out to best male friend ($.18, p < .01$), out to academic advisor ($.18, p < .05$), and out to mother ($.15, p < .05$). Correlations between self-esteem and out to father ($.03$), sibling ($.04$), and best female friend ($.13$) were not significant. The Openness factor accounted for a significant portion of the variance in predicting level of self-esteem among the males. Although self-esteem was significantly correlated with general openness ($.23, p < .05$) among the lesbians, none of the other correlations (ranging from $.06$ to $-.09$) was significant. The lesbian model was not significant when both the General/Family Openness and Open to Friends factors were placed in the regression model (Table 7.7).

DISCUSSION

Disclosure of oneself as a lesbian or gay person to self and others is, in most respects, a complex process (Fitzpatrick, 1983). To divide, subdivide, delineate, and then attempt to define stages or sequences of the coming-out process is, at the level of the individual undergoing the process, somewhat artificial. In this respect it is similar to many other psychosocial dynamics that an individual experiences. Thus, any effort to research this issue must, by necessity, be cautious and sensitive to diversity across and within individuals.

Unfortunately, however, the coming-out literature reviewed in this chapter seems firmly committed to a stage model perspective. Thus, the internal cognitive and psychodynamic dimensions of feeling different, self-recognition, and self-acceptance are viewed in conjunction with external manifestations of disclosure to others. But how do they "fit" together? If many gay males and lesbians are "doing" before "being," they have "disclosed" to their sexual partners and perhaps their associates and outside viewers their sexual orientation without any conscious self-recognition or self-acceptance of being homosexual. On the other hand, one may know and accept one's homosexuality, not disclose that information to any or few others, and still lead a healthy, fulfilling life.

Table 7.7 Regression predicting self-esteem from Openness factor for males and females

Source	Full model					Parameter estimates			
	df	M^2	F	p	r^2	df	SE	t	p
Males									
Model	1	159.31	5.40	.02	.04				
Error	119	29.49							
Factor									
Openness						1	.50	2.32	.02
Females									
Model	2	1.66	.08	.93	.00				
Error	54	21.33							
Factor									
General/Family Openness						1	.66	.06	.96
Open to Friends						1	.65	.35	.73

In an attempt to avoid some of the difficulties noted above, in this research project I bypassed an entire meaning of coming out: the experiential dimension regarding self-conception and self-definition. In large part this was necessitated by the methodology adopted in the current research, one that is inadequate to assess aspects of the "identity" process in a coming-out definition. A more in-depth instrument, such as an interview technique, would be necessary to explore dimensions of awareness, feelings, and acceptance.[4] The focus here is on the disclosure dimension, including both passing and being known about.

Coming out was defined as the extent to which one believes that others know that he or she is gay or lesbian. Usually, when an individual states that he or she is out, additional issues must be raised: To whom? Who was first? How many know? The target of disclosure is critical because an individual generally does not come out to all others at the same time, especially initially when a gay or lesbian youth is quite selective in terms of disclosure. Important is the relationship the youth has with the target person and the expected reaction of the person to the new information. If the target person is viewed as warm, accepting, and nurturant and thus supportive of the adolescent as an individual, then the likelihood of the youth's coming out to that person is great. Usually the information is not totally new; the target may have suspected that the youth's sexual orientation was not heterosexual. These latter issues are addressed insofar as they relate to family relationships in Chapter 8.

For the male youths in the current sample there appeared to be only one disclosure variable; if a youth was out to one individual then he was out to everyone. This does not imply, however, the absence of a rank order of disclosure. It appeared that male youths generally told a close peer or peers before family members and mothers before fathers. Disclosure to these classes of individuals and being out to everyone were correlated with positive self-esteem.

The last finding was replicated with the female youths. On the other hand, all correlations among the disclosure categories were not significant, especially when academic advisor was one of the categories. The rank order of telling others would

---

[4]These data are currently being collected with gay youths.

appear to be similar to that of the males with two notable exceptions: Siblings were told earlier and fathers were generally the last to know. These results support other research (Bender et al., 1976; McKirnan & Peterson, 1986) that found gay males and lesbians disclose first to close friends rather than to parents.

There can be little doubt that disclosure to others varies among individuals. Researchers have devoted some attention not only to distinguishing characteristics of those one comes out to but also to describing those who are out and those who are not. Few of these studies address characteristics of adolescents and youth. The results from the present investigation are contrasted below with the adult literature, noting similarities that appear not to be age bound, as well as age-specific findings.

The best predictors of whether a lesbian or gay youth in the current study was publicly out were factors in the gay-related activity cluster of variables. For both lesbians and gay males the Activism factor was the single best predictor: Those most out actively participated in gay rights activities, socialized with other lesbians and gays, attended lesbian and gay activities, and read lesbian and gay periodicals. Congruent with several other research findings, those most out held positive views of their sexual orientation and would not give it up even if they could. This does not support the no-relationship result between the two variables reported by others (e.g., Harry & DeVall, 1978).

These findings counter the view that by coming out one becomes alienated from the lesbian and gay communities; clearly, coming out and participating in the lesbian and gay communities were related for the youths in this study. Disclosure and involvement in the lesbian and gay communities were closely linked, as they have been in the vast majority of adult studies. Perhaps in some sense these gay-related activities define disclosure; they are probably both antecedents and consequences of coming out of the closet.

There were also several differences between gay males and lesbians that are worth noting. Male youths who were out had felt their sexual orientation at an early age, believed their homosexuality was beyond their control, frequently went to gay bars, and had had many homosexual sexual encounters. Lesbians who had had few heterosexual sexual experiences, who had felt their sexual orientation at an early age, and who believed they had little choice in being a lesbian were most likely to publicly disclose their homosexuality. Thus, recognizing one's homosexuality at an early age and believing one had little control in determining that sexual orientation were advantages for the youths in terms of coming out. For the lesbians the former finding is somewhat inconsistent with Elliot's (1982) research. Among males these issues have been generally ignored by investigators.

Harry and DeVall (1978) reported that the earlier a gay male came out the more likely he was to engage in early homosexual sex. The male youths in the present study confirmed this: The more out an individual was, the more likely he was to engage in homosexual sex and to patronize a gay bar.

Where a youth placed himself or herself on the homosexual–heterosexual continuum was not predictive of public disclosure. This is counter to several investigators of adults (e.g., Bell & Weinberg, 1978; McDonald, 1982). In partial support, however, out lesbians had had few heterosexual sexual experiences and out gay males had had many homosexual sexual experiences.

For both lesbian and gay youths, the second most important cluster of variables was the same: Support from Family and Friends. The sexes diverged somewhat in the relative importance of family and friends. For lesbians, acceptance from family members accounted for the vast proportion of the variance within the model; reporting a large number of gay and lesbian friends was secondary. Among the male youths, however, acceptance from friends was clearly most crucial in coming out; acceptance from mother and closest sibling was secondary. A large number of homosexual and heterosexual friends approached significance for the males. In a global sense these results are consistent with the scant adult literature that indicates that having supportive, accepting friends and relatives is more important than the absolute number of friends. In addition, whereas having a large number of straight friends was important for a gay male to come out, for a lesbian it was more important to have friends, regardless of gender, of the same sexual orientation. These gender differences, are relatively undocumented in the literature and are further explored in Chapters 8 and 9.

Most adult studies ignore aspects of personality and self-worth when distinguishing those who are out from those who are not. Data from the lesbian youths in the present study appear to justify this omission: Only one self-assessment factor was significantly related to disclosure. On the other hand, gay youths who were most out described themselves as accomplished and self-sufficient; those not out were most likely to report themselves as compassionate, expressive of tender feelings easily, affectionate, aggressive, forceful, and competitive. Close male and female friends were important as were material possessions and a high frequency of sex, to the self-worth of nondisclosing male youths. These results indicate that future research should explore the personality profiles of gay males who are and are not out. Those not out may be of at least two types: the very "feminine" and the very "masculine."

Love affair variables were not predictive of coming out among the gay males in the study. But among females, those whose first love affair had been homosexual and who had a high percentage of homosexual rather than heterosexual love affairs were most likely to disclose to others. There is scant empirical research on adults with which to compare these findings. The current results support McKirnan and Peterson's finding that being in a current relationship was relatively unimportant for degree of outness (P. Peterson, personal communication, 1988). Harry and DeVall (1978) indicated that among gay men coming out was significantly correlated with having homosexual love affairs during adolescence. Support for this finding in the present study was not provided by the gay males but by the lesbian youths.

Although prior research has generally ignored age trends in disclosure within adolescent populations, the logic of coming-out stage models that places disclosure to others as a late event implies that with age there is a corresponding increase in coming out. Studies with adults usually support this projection. The present research confirmed this for the male but not the female youths. Male youths most out were also the oldest, had the most years of education, and had physically matured early. The last finding is intriguing. Perhaps the early maturation of one's biological self, including erotic attractions, brings with it early awareness of homosexual feelings and thus recognition of one's homosexuality. None of these relationships was significant for the females, which is somewhat puzzling. If, in fact, the critical coming-out ages for lesbians are later than for males, then a wider range and diversity of coming-out experiences among lesbians would have been included had the age limit been extended in this research, and the results found here might have duplicated the male data. In actuality, the lesbians were more out than were the males.

Social class status did not predict coming out among the females, but it approached significance for the males. Consistent with the empirical literature (except for McKirnan & Peterson, 1986), gay males from upper income homes were more likely to be out to others. Prior research has also indicated that growing up in larger urban areas is more conducive to coming out because of its anonymity. On this point the lesbians confirmed the research; findings for the gay males were in the same direction but not significant.

Males who were liberal and pro-feminism were most likely to be out. Issues of political and social ideology are seldom addressed in the coming-out empirical literature. Degree of religiosity, counter to the literature, was relatively unrelated to homosexual disclosure. Cohort effects may be important here. On the whole, the youths in the present study were not particularly attracted to religious institutions (a large number of "none"s in religious affiliation) or religious feelings. Thus, they may have been relatively insulated, compared with adults in other studies, from the generally negative, homophobic views of religion.

Two primary questions emerge when considering issues of disclosure and psychological well-being: Are the two related, and if so, what is the cause–effect relationship between the two? The empirical literature appears to converge on the conclusion that whereas the psychological aspects of coming out (i.e., self-recognition and self-acceptance) are positively related to self-esteem, disclosure to others is less frequently a significant predictor of self-worth variables. Psychologists (e.g., Malyon, 1981) tend to view a positive sense of self as leading to progressive coming-out developments, whereas sociologists (e.g., Weinberg & Williams, 1974) view the process in reverse: By coming out men and women are more likely to accept themselves and their homosexual orientation. There is clearly a cost, however, to publicly coming out: increased personal harassment, verbal abuse, assault, institutional discrimination, and discrimination from other lesbians and gay men (McKirnan & Peterson, 1987a). Although these instances led to increased levels of stress, they did not generally affect the self-image of lesbians and gay men in Chicago.

Few of the studies cited here addressed these issues with youths. Malyon (1981) believed that although disclosure of one's homosexuality is generally a positive developmental asset during adolescence, enhancing crisis competence, self-respect, and ego integrity, "for the individual who opts for a homosexual identity during adolescence, many problems complicate and interfere with a desirable outcome to the developmental process. Social attitudes militate against feelings of self-acceptance" (p. 328). The findings for the gay youths reported in this chapter do not support this last assertion; nor do they support the no-difference results of Weinberg and Williams (1974). Rather, males who were most out of the closet to others reported the highest levels of self-esteem. Apparently, when gay youths evaluated themselves as positive and worthwhile persons it was not dependent on the hostile social world in which they live. If they had ever experienced the ongoing negative attitude of others toward homosexuality they either did not internalize it as a statement about the self or they had the necessary coping resources to overcome the negativity. These findings leave unaddressed the issue of causation— whether psychological health led to disclosure to others, or whether by disclosing to others higher levels of self-esteem were achieved.

In contrast, disclosure to others was not predicted by self-esteem level among the lesbian youths. This finding is consistent with the results of other studies (Elliot, 1982; Sanders, 1980) and of the rest of the present research, which indicates that lesbian self-esteem is not as predicated on the variables tested as is male self-esteem level. One must search elsewhere for correlates of lesbian self-esteem. Relationship with parents is explored in Chapter 8. A more general overview of gender difference is pursued in Chapter 9.

8

The Significance of Parents for Coming Out and Self-Esteem

OVERVIEW

The variables that were used to predict self-esteem and coming out were reapplied to focus specifically on the youths' relationships with the parents. Two models have been frequently used to describe the parent–youth interpersonal dynamic. The first, reflected appraisals, is a popular sociological theory, and the second, a coming-out-right perspective, has wide clinical appeal.

In the study of the reflected appraisals perspective, the emphasis was on the importance of the parents for the youth's well-being, especially the variables youth's comfortableness with her or his sexual orientation and parents' acceptance of their offspring's sexual orientation. In the second part of the study, the coming-out-right advice literature, which is nearly uniform in underscoring the significance of the parents for the young lesbian's or gay male's sense of self, was examined. Variables studied from this perspective were age and marital status of the parents, the youth's satisfaction and contact with her or his parents, and the parents' knowledge of their child's homosexuality.

REFLECTED APPRAISALS[1]

Literature

In American society it is axiomatic that we are a social species, responding almost without recourse to the attitudes and actions of others in the environment. A sociological perspective, reflected appraisals, that was introduced in Chapter 2, is a manifestation of this view:

> *Reduced to essentials, the principle holds that people, as social animals, are deeply influenced by the attitudes of others toward the self and that, in the course of time, they come to view themselves as they are viewed by others. (Rosenberg, 1979, p. 63)*

The present research focused on one aspect of that social environment, family relations, with the goal of determining the degree to which parents' attitudes toward their son's or daughter's sexual orientation, as perceived by the youth, affect the youth's comfortableness with that sexual orientation and, in turn, his or her level of self-esteem.

As articulated by Rosenberg (1979), the reflected appraisals model assumes three interrelated principles:

[1]This section is based on an earlier report of these data (Savin-Williams, 1989a).

1. Our conception and evaluation of the self is largely formed by the responses of others to us. Because we seek "consensual validation" of our self-concepts, we test ourselves within a social context. Through the process of communication, we experience the self not directly but indirectly by taking the role of others, ultimately adopting their attitudes toward us.

2. This conception is not a literal, mechanical transformation of others' attitudes; more important is how we believe we appear to others. How we imagine that we are judged by others in the social world is influential in affecting our conceptions and evaluations of the self. Cooley's (1912) term for this phenomenon was the "looking-glass self".[2]

3. Our "self-concept is shaped by the attitudes of others, not as a direct reflection of these attitudes, but by applying to the self the attitudes of the society as a whole" (Rosenberg, 1979, p. 67). Through social processes and experiences we come to recognize the attitudes of the generalized other, the sum of the many attitudes toward us. Thus, as noted by Weinberg (1983), the feelings that gay people have about themselves are intimately related to their perception of the feedback that they receive from others.

In his classical "revelation" of the gay world, Hoffman (1968) maintained that low self-esteem among male homosexuals is the result of an acceptance of the verdict made by a homophobic culture that homosexuality is immoral, psychologically sick, and a crime. These values and attitudes, especially among parents, siblings, and teachers, were prevalent as the gay or lesbian person grew up. The assumed and thus encouraged norm was heterosexuality. Homosexuality was either invisible to the individual or condemned. This message, given to the child, was later accepted by the adolescent and the adult. As a result, the gay person's self-evaluation suffered. One need not experience the negative reaction directly (such as being called "faggot"); the imagined fear of a negative sanction is sometimes more powerful than an actual assault on one's self-image (Weinberg & Williams, 1974).

Perhaps most critical for the evolving sense of self is the family. A number of investigators have documented the importance of family relations in influencing an adolescent's self-esteem (Demo, Small, & Savin-Williams, 1987; Gecas & Schwalbe, 1986; Openshaw, Thomas, & Rollins, 1984). Consistent with Cooley's (1912) principle of the looking-glass self, it is not so much the actual attitudes of the parents that influence the development and maintenance of an adolescent's self-evaluation as it is the youth's perception of the parents' attitudes. For example, Demo et al. (1987) discovered that the self-esteem of both male and female adolescents was best predicted by their reports of parent–adolescent communications and not by the parents' reports of whether they communicated well with their adolescent children (which explained little of the variance in an adolescent's self-evaluation). Thus, to understand a youth's image of herself or himself it is more important to examine the attitudes that the youth believes the parents have toward

[2]This restriction omits two other dimensions of the reflected appraisals perspective: direct reflections and the generalized other (Rosenberg, 1979, p. 63). Direct reflections refer "to how particular others view us" and its omission is discussed in the text; the second, the generalized other which refers "to the attitudes of the community as a whole," is not examined because of the developmental rather than sociological orientation of this book.

him or her and how important those attitudes are for his or her sense of self than to examine the parents' actual attitudes toward the youth.

Rosenberg (1979, p. 83) noted, "Not all significant others are equally significant, and those who are more significant have greater influence on our self-concepts." Although one often assumes that parents are significant for an adolescent's self-esteem, this is an empirical question. In the present study this assumption was tested by asking the study participants, "How important is your relationship with your parents to your sense of self-worth?" The responses were integrated into a model predicting self-esteem level.

On the basis of a reflected appraisals perspective, the following model is proposed. For lesbian and gay youths who view the parents as an important aspect of their sense of self-worth, the degree to which they also report that the parents have accepted (or would accept if they knew) their homosexuality will determine whether the youths will feel comfortable with their sexual orientation. The greater the perceived acceptance rather than rejection, the less likely the adolescents will want to give up their homosexuality. Because relationships with parents are not always equal, this hypothesis was examined separately for mother and father. Finally, it is proposed that the more youths feel comfortable with their sexual orientation, the higher will be their level of self-esteem. Although there was little reason to expect the genders to differ in fulfilling the reflected appraisals model, analyses were conducted separately for the lesbian and gay youths.

Present Study Methods

Comfortableness

Two questions from the Gay and Lesbian Questionnaire (GAL Q) were summed for the dimension of comfortableness in being gay or lesbian. These were "I would not give up my homosexuality even if I could" and "I feel my life would be much easier if I were heterosexual." Responses for each ranged from 1 (*strongly disagree*) to 9 (*strongly agree*). Respondents' answers were combined after reversing scores on the second question. On the basis of a sample of 19, the combined reliability coefficient was .65.

Parental Acceptance

Each adolescent was asked on the GAL Q, "How has your mother/father reacted (or how do you think she or he would react) to the fact that you are gay?" The 4-point continuum included the options *accepting (or it would not matter), tolerant (but not accepting), intolerant (but not rejecting),* and *rejecting.* The reliability scores for mother and father were .58.

Parental Importance

On a scale of 1 to 9, the youths rated how important their parents were to their sense of self-worth. The continuum ranged from *extremely not important* (1) to *extremely important* (9). Test–retest reliability was .86.

Data Analysis

Standard least-squares regression analyses were computed for each sex separately (omitting missing data cases for each analysis), for mother variables, and for father variables. In the first series of regressions, comfortableness was the dependent variable and mother or father acceptance was the independent variable. Next, importance and its interaction with acceptance were placed in the model to test for the significance of the parental relationship.

In the self-esteem regression analyses both comfortableness and mother or father acceptance were inserted as independent variables, separate for each sex and for each parent. Finally, importance and its interactions with both comfortableness and acceptance were added to the model.

Present Study Results

Descriptive Data

On the 9-point comfortableness scale, the males were at the midpoint (4.40). The females were somewhat more likely to report comfortableness with their sexual orientation (3.67). The difference was apparent not so much in response to the question "I feel my life would be easier if I were heterosexual," as in the desire to give up their homosexuality if they could (males were 1 point higher).

Mothers were perceived by the gay youths as more accepting and less rejecting of their son's homosexuality than were fathers (see Table 6.19). Thirty-two percent of the mothers were reported to be accepting and only 10% were seen as rejecting; among fathers the percentages were 23% and 22%, respectively. Among lesbians, mothers and fathers were equally perceived to be accepting/rejecting (see Table 6.22): 25% and 23%, respectively (accepting) and 17% and 18%, respectively (rejecting). Thus, gay and lesbian youths held similar views regarding the acceptance and rejection they received from their fathers but lesbians were more likely than gay males to report lower levels of acceptance and higher levels of rejection from their mothers. Lesbians were slightly more likely to perceive that the parents were important for their sense of self-worth ($M = 3.02$ and 3.27, respectively).

Predicting Comfortableness

The expectation that if the parents accepted their child's homosexuality then the adolescent should feel comfortable being lesbian or gay was confirmed for females but not for males, as shown in Table 8.1.

This relationship was expected to be stronger when the importance of the parent was considered: The more significant the parents are perceived to be for one's sense of self-worth, the greater should be their impact on one's comfortableness with being gay or lesbian and one's self-esteem level. Adding importance and its interaction effects with mother acceptance, however, contributed little to the prediction of a lesbian's comfortableness with her homosexuality (increasing the attributed variance to 7%), although they had the expected effect (increasing explained variance to 11%) with father acceptance. The correlation between father

Table 8.1 Predicting comfortableness with being homosexual for male and female youths on the basis of their perceptions of mother and father acceptance

Acceptance	df, n	M^2	% explained variance	F	p
Males					
Mother	1, 198	2.60	1	.59	.445
Father	1, 192	.51	1	.12	.733
Females					
Mother	1, 96	18.65	5	5.35	.023
Father	1, 92	24.47	6	7.22	.009

acceptance and comfortableness was considerably higher for lesbians who reported that their parents were important components of their self-worth (.33, $p = .003$) than for those who maintained that the parents were relatively unimportant (.03, NS).

Adding importance strengthened both the mother acceptance and the father acceptance models among gay youths to a level of significantly predicting the males' comfortableness being gay, $F(3, 195) = 3.19, p = .02$, and $F(3, 189) = 2.90, p = .03$, respectively. The correlations between mother acceptance and comfortableness and father acceptance and comfortableness were higher for males who reported that the parents were important ($r = .14, p = .09$, and $r = .11, p = .18$, respectively) rather than unimportant ($r = .04$, NS, and $r = -.14$, NS, respectively) for their sense of self.

Predicting Self-Esteem

It was hypothesized that self-esteem would be highest among youths who felt most comfortable with their homosexuality because the parents, an important aspect of their social and interpersonal world, accepted their sexual orientation. For the lesbians this was clearly not the case (Table 8.2), for either the mother acceptance or father acceptance model. Adding importance and its interactions did little in the maternal model but it increased the amount of variance accounted for in the paternal model to 6%, $F(5, 86) = 2.24, p = .057$. That is, for females who reported that the parents were a significant influence for their sense of self-worth, the positive relationship between father acceptance and self-esteem approached statistical significance, $t(1) = 1.83, p = .07$.

For gay males, however, the models were strongly confirmed (Table 8.2), primarily because feeling comfortable with one's homosexuality and self-esteem were highly interrelated. Adding importance and its interactions had relatively little impact on the results except to mediate mother and father acceptance. Thus, the direct effect of mother and father acceptance on self-esteem was reduced to nonsignificance when importance was added to the models because of the high correlations between importance and acceptance variables: For mother acceptance, $t(1) = 1.47, p = .14$; for father acceptance, $t(1) = 1.33, p = .19$.

Table 8.2 Predicting self-esteem among gay and lesbian youths from the dimensions comfortableness with being homosexual and parental acceptance

Dimension	df, n	M^2	% of explained variance	F	p	df	t	p
			Males					
Mother	2, 195	268.19	10	10.64				
Acceptance						1	2.00	.047
Comfortableness						1	4.03	.0001
Father	2, 190	243.83	9	9.45				
Acceptance						1	1.62	.106
Comfortableness						1	3.99	.0001
			Females					
Mother	2, 93	12.31	1	.58				
Acceptance						1	.53	.600
Comfortableness						1	.81	.419
Father	2, 89	28.77	3	1.40				
Acceptance						1	1.14	.259
Comfortableness						1	.90	.368

The header of the table includes a spanning "Full model" over df,n / M^2 / % of explained variance / F / p, and "Parameter estimates" over df / t / p.

COMING OUT RIGHT TO PARENTS[3]

Literature

For many gay and lesbian youths the most difficult decision to make after recognizing and then accepting to some degree their nontraditional sexual orientation is to reveal to their parents that they will not be fulfilling the heterosexual dreams of the parents. This appears intuitively obvious, and, indeed, coming-out-right advice books strongly emphasize the critical importance of the parents in the coming-out process. On the other hand, theoretical models (see Chapter 3) that describe the coming-out process have largely ignored the role that the parents have on this dimension of their child's development. The first section of this chapter confirmed aspects of the coming-out-right literature by reporting on the relationships among the parents' reaction (or how they would react if they knew) to the knowledge of their son's or daughter's homosexuality, the importance of the parents for a youth's sense of self-worth, the youth's comfortableness being lesbian or gay, and his or her self-esteem level. This section extends the investigation by examining (a) characteristics of the parents and their relationship with the youth that influence the parents' knowledge of the youth's sexual orientation and (b) how these in combination affect the youth's self-esteem level.

The self-help advice literature explicitly highlights the significance of parents for youths' coming-out process and self-evaluation. According to this perspective,

---

[3]This section is based on an earlier report of these data (Savin-Williams, 1989b).

some gay males and lesbians never come out to their parents, becoming, according to MacDonald (1983),

> half-members of the family unit, afraid and alienated, unable ever to be totally open and spontaneous, to trust or be trusted, to develop a fully socialized sense of self affirmation. This sad stunting of human potential breeds stress for gay people and their families alike—stress characterized by secrecy, ignorance, helplessness, and distance. (p. 1)

Under such conditions youths may respond by running away from home or by becoming involved in prostitution or other crimes. They may feel that they are unable to cope with the obligatory deception, isolation, and alienation (Clark, 1977; Martin, 1982).

Gay teenagers have given first-person accounts of the emotional significance and danger of coming out to parents. Heron (1983) has collected some of these in *One Teenager in Ten*:

> Perhaps nothing is riskier than coming out to parents. I came out to my parents at the same time I came out to myself, but I wasn't prepared for their reaction. . . . "You can't be gay! You must be mistaken." They were so upset they sent me back to school and said, "Don't come back home until we say you can." Those were the most painful words I've ever heard. For a brief moment I considered suicide, but I had friends and ministers to turn to for support. I was not alone. (Rick, p. 97)

> I also told my father. The one phrase that I'll remember is, "Your mother and I have no further reason to live. I don't know what the hell we have done to deserve the treatment we are getting. Terry, you were our only hope." (Terry, p. 73)

In books written to assist gay and lesbian individuals to develop in a healthy manner there is a careful, considered approach to the issue of revealing sexual orientation to parents. Gains and losses must be balanced because parents have the capacity and power to inflict ostracism, rejection, isolation, and even violence (Muchmore & Hanson, 1982; Silverstein, 1977). Generally, parents should not be told unless the youth has developed a relatively secure, positive view of homosexuality and has a good relationship with the parents (Silverstein, 1977).

Given the historical condemnation of homosexuality and the tendency for most parents to consider their children to be extensions of themselves, Weinberg (1972) observed that for many gay youth difficulties with parents are profoundly significant. Telling parents may be the final exit out of the closet. Fairchild and Hayward's (1979) book, as well as others (Berzon & Leighton, 1979; Borhek, 1983; Clark, 1977; Silverstein, 1977; Woodman & Lenna, 1980), suggest strategies for parents who need help in coping with the seemingly earth-shattering news of their child's homosexuality.

The most accurate generalization that can be made, however, is that the reaction of parents to the news appears "unpredictable" (Borhek, 1983), although most writers believe that a positive prior relationship with the parents is a good omen for a healthy resolution (Borhek, 1983; Fairchild & Hayward, 1979; Silverstein, 1977; Weinberg, 1972). Having elderly parents may be a bad omen. They may have difficulty accepting their child's homosexuality because of the social and political climate of their child-rearing years (e.g., McCarthy era) when homosexuality was viewed as an unspeakable, moral sin or a deep, psychological pathology (Borhek, 1983).

The advice literature is less clearly unanimous on the effects that coming out to parents has on the self-evaluations of gay males and lesbians. If the consequences are affirming and supportive, Borhek (1983) believes, then telling will enhance self-esteem because "You may have a clearer sense of your identity and a new sense of freedom and self-respect because now you are not hiding your real self" (p. 20). Both parents and youth can prosper because by coming out one is able to "share joyfully and with a sense of well-being with the significant persons in your life because you have taken the positive step of being real with them" (p. 20).

Theoretical and Empirical Literature

In contrast to this high priority on the parent–child relationship during the youth's revelatory process, the theoretical and empirical coming-out literature largely ignores or deemphasizes the issue (Cass, 1979, 1984; Dank, 1971, 1973; de Monteflores & Schultz, 1978; Lee, 1977; McDonald, 1982; Myrick, 1974a, 1974b; Plummer, 1975; Schafer, 1977; Troiden, 1979, 1989; Weinberg, 1978). Troiden (1989) noted that an accepting family is one of several facilitating factors in the coming-out process; Myrick (1974a, 1974b) included "out to family" with being out to employer, future employer, male acquaintance, and best heterosexual friend in his measure of self-disclosure. Cass (1979) treated parents as one aspect of a category that included peers, church group, and heterosexuals in general as a determining factor in whether an individual will "pass" as a heterosexual or come out. Coleman (1982) noted the significance of telling parents, but stated that one should first gauge whether the parents will be accepting.

Gay males and lesbians usually reveal their sexual orientation first to close friends (Hencken, 1985; also see Chapter 6). The nuclear family is generally told fairly soon thereafter, although there is relatively little empirical research on the factors that determine whether adolescents will reveal their homosexuality to the parents or on the effects that coming out to parents has on a youth's self-esteem. In general, one is more likely to come out to mother than to father and other family members (Cohen-Ross, 1985; Cramer, 1986; Grabert, 1985; Remafedi, 1987a; also see Chapter 6). In a West German sample of lesbians (Schafer, 1976), 44% were out to mother and 32% to father; in a San Francisco Bay Area sample of White homosexual persons (Bell & Weinberg, 1978), 42% of males and 49% of females were out to mother and 31% of males and 37% of females were out to father. The difference is usually attributable to the fact that mothers are more likely to respond in an affirming manner (Jay & Young, 1979). For example, in Remafedi's (1987a) sample of 29 bisexual and gay teenagers, 62% were out to their mothers but only 34% were out to fathers. Far more (93%) had told a friend. The mothers were more likely than fathers to respond positively (21% vs. 10%) to the news; negative reactions to the revelation were the norm, however, for both parents.

Many never come out to their parents, even as adults, because of the fear that such disclosure would have negative implications for their relationship with the parents or their status within the family. There may also be anxiety that the news will hurt their parents (Cramer, 1986; Koodin et al., 1979). Several studies (Bell &

Weinberg, 1978; Jay & Young, 1979) reported that more than one-half of the sampled population had not told parents of their sexual orientation.

The dissertation research of Cramer (1986) confirmed many of these findings. He gave a questionnaire to various gay organizations and discovered that the 93 male respondents were more likely to be out to mother (63%) than to father (59%) and that more mothers than fathers were told directly, rather than indirectly. The men reported that their relationship with their mother was more positive than with their father, but this was true regardless of whether they were out or closeted. Although the parent–son relationship deteriorated immediately after disclosure, it improved considerably thereafter. Contrary to other reports, the initial reactions of the mothers were more negative than those the fathers displayed, and relations with fathers improved more than they did with the mothers. Perhaps most revealing, more nondisclosers feared the reactions of their father (70%) than feared the reactions of their mother (61%).

Cramer (1986) also found that those who disclosed to the parents had significantly high levels of self-esteem. Other significant predictors of self-esteem were current positive parental relationship and length of time one has been out to the parents (although this might be confounded by the age of the subject). The initial reaction of the parents was unrelated to the son's self-esteem score. In the Bell and Weinberg (1978) sample, self-acceptance was highest among adult gay men who were most likely to be out to their parents (functionals and close-coupleds) and lowest among those least likely to be out to parents (dysfunctionals and asexuals). No such trend was evident among the women.

As noted earlier, in the present study the average lesbian felt most comfortable with her sexual orientation if she also reported that her parents accepted or would accept if they knew her sexual orientation. Their perceived acceptance did not, however, predict her level of self-esteem. Among males, parental acceptance was related to feeling comfortable being gay if the youths also reported that the parents were important to their sense of self-worth; males comfortable with their sexual orientation had positive self-esteem.

On the basis of the analyses of the data reported earlier in this chapter and the coming-out-right advice literature, there is sufficient reason to believe that parents are a significant factor in their child's developing sense of self-worth and sexual identity, especially in terms of the youth's feeling comfortable with her or his homosexuality and of the youth's disclosing that information to others. The theoretical coming-out literature, however, appears to contradict these assertions by essentially ignoring the role of the parents in the coming-out process. The present research attempted to bridge these two literatures by proposing that the following variables would increase the probability that the parents know the sexual orientation of their child:[4]

1. The adolescent reports satisfaction and contact with the parent,
2. The parents are married rather than separated or divorced,
3. The parents are young rather than old.

---

[4]These variables were selected rather than "importance of the parents for one's sense of self-worth" because the coming-out advice literature does not question this relationship; it assumes they are intimately related. The correlations of these four variables with importance ranged from .19 to .44 for lesbians and .23 to .47 for gay males. Thus, although there is much overlap, there is also considerable independence among these variables.

In addition, these variables were expected to predict positive self-esteem for the adolescent. Because of the possibility that these relationships are dependent on the sex of the adolescent and/or the parent, all analyses were conducted separately for gay males and lesbians and for fathers and mothers.

Present Study Methods

Parents' Knowledge of Their Child's Homosexuality

In response to the GAL Q question "Do the following people know that you are gay?", each youth indicated one of four responses: *definitely knows and we have talked about it, definitely knows but we have never talked about it, probably knows or suspects,* or *does not know or suspect.* Included in the list of people were mother and father. This variable was the youth's knowledge of whether or not the parent knew (see Chapter 4 for reliability data).

Satisfaction With Maternal and Paternal Relationship

On a scale from *extremely satisfied* (1) to *not at all satisfied* (9), each youth answered the question "How satisfied are you with your relationship with your parents?" Mother and father were assessed separately. On the basis of the sample of 19, test–retest reliabilities were .92 for maternal and .75 for paternal satisfaction.

Contact With Parents

One of nine categories was selected by the youths in response to the question "Overall, how often do you have any kind of contact (by phone, mail, visits, etc.) with your mother/father?" The range was from *daily to almost everyday* (1) to *once a month* (5) to *never* (9). Reliability coefficients were .78 for contact with mother and .75 for contact with father.

Parents' Marital Status

The youths indicated if their biological parents were currently married, separated, or divorced. Test–retest scores were all identical.

Age of Parents

From the GAL Q question "How old are your parents?", the ages of the mother and father were assessed. Reliability coefficients were .88 for mother and .96 for father.

Data Analysis

Data analyses proceeded in four steps:

1. Descriptive accounts of the dependent and independent variables;
2. Correlations of the study's variables;
3. Regression of the independent variables on parents' knowledge of their son's or daughter's homosexuality;
4. Regression of the above variables on the self-esteem of the youths.

Regression procedures were standard, least-squares linear regressions.

Present Study Results

Descriptive Data

Table 8.3 presents the raw data and means for all variables: youth's satisfaction and contact with their parents, parents' marital status, and parents' age. In general, there were relatively few differences between gay and lesbian youths. The vast majority, 77% of the males and 66% of the females, grew up in homes in which both parents were present and married to each other. Females were slightly more satisfied than males with their relationships with the parents, but they had less contact with parents than did males. Gay males were more out to their fathers than lesbians were to their fathers.

As might be expected, mothers were younger ($M = 49$ years old) than fathers ($M = 51$ years old) and the youths reported greater satisfaction and more contact with mothers. More than one-third of all youths reported very bad relationships with their father; with mother, 15%. At least weekly contact with mother was characteristic of 53% of the lesbians and 58% of the gay males; comparable percentages with father were 33% and 42%, respectively. Fathers were less likely to know of their child's sexual orientation than were mothers. Overall, 34% of the youths reported that their father did not know of their sexual orientation, and 24% reported that their mother did not know.

Table 8.4 presents the correlations of these variables for the lesbians. There was high congruency in the data lesbians reported for mothers and fathers on the same dimension. Thus, if mother knew, father knew; on the average, if the lesbian youth was satisfied with her relationship with mother and had frequent contact with her, then she was also satisfied with her paternal relationship and had frequent contact with her father. The ages of the parents were highly correlated with each other.

Contact with a parent was highly related to reported satisfaction with that parent. Daughters with married parents reported more contact and greater satisfaction with their father than daughters from divorced or separated homes. If the parents were married, they were more likely to be of an advanced age.

Young mothers and fathers were most likely to know that their daughter was a lesbian. In addition, lesbians who reported that their father knew their sexual orientation were most likely to report a good relationship with him. Only two variables were significantly correlated with a lesbian's self-esteem: having a young mother and being satisfied with the maternal relationship. These two were not, however, highly correlated with each other.

The data for the gay youths are presented in Table 8.5. Similar to results obtained from the lesbian youths, all mother–father comparable data (knows, contact, satisfaction, age) were significantly correlated with each other.

Contact with father was significantly correlated with male youths' reports of satisfaction with their relationship; a similar trend ($p = .07$) was found for mother. Gay males expressed better relationships with young mothers than with older ones, and they had more contact with married than with divorced or separated parents.

Table 8.3 Frequency and percentage of responses for independent variables for male and female youths in the coming-out-right analysis

Variable	Frequency[a]		% of responses	
	Males	Females	Males	Females
Satisfaction with father				
1 (High)	13	5	7	5
2	20	12	10	13
3	24	16	12	17
4	15	6	8	6
5	24	9	12	9
6	30	14	15	15
7	29	10	15	10
8	24	16	12	17
9 (Low)	21	8	11	8
M	5.37	5.24		
Satisfaction with mother				
1 (High)	27	13	13	13
2	37	18	18	18
3	41	24	20	24
4	28	14	14	14
5	23	5	11	5
6	23	8	11	8
7	10	8	5	8
8	12	7	6	7
9 (Low)	6	3	3	3
M	3.98	3.92		
Contact with father				
1 (Frequent)	22	5	11	5
2	9	5	4	5
3	54	22	26	23
4	66	38	32	39
5	23	11	11	11
6	18	13	9	13
7	4	1	2	1
8	2	1	1	1
9 (Infrequent)	6	1	3	1
M	3.84	4.04		
Contact with mother				
1 (Frequent)	28	8	13	8
2	16	7	8	7
3	78	38	37	38
4	59	36	28	36
5	15	8	7	8
6	10	2	5	2
7	1	0	1	0
8	0	1	0	1
9 (Infrequent)	2	0	1	0
M	3.32	3.40		
Parents married				
Yes	166	68	79	67
No	44	34	21	33
Father's age				
30s	8	4	4	4
40s	75	35	38	36

Table 8.3   (Continued)

Variable	Frequency[a]		% of responses	
	Males	Females	Males	Females
Father's age (continued)				
50s	91	48	46	49
60s +	26	10	13	10
M	51.36	51.06		
Mother's age				
30s	13	6	6	6
40s	101	50	49	51
50s	78	36	38	36
60s +	13	7	6	7
M	48.74	48.57		
Father knows				
1 (Yes)	80	26	40	26
2	11	16	5	16
3	46	17	23	18
4 (No)	65	38	32	39
M	2.41	2.71		
Mother knows				
1 (Yes)	98	47	47	47
2	16	13	8	13
3	42	20	20	20
4 (No)	53	20	25	20
M	2.15	2.14		
Self-esteem				
Range	8–30	10–30		
M	21.98	22.18		

[a]Excluding missing data.

On the average, a male with high self-esteem level reported satisfying relationships with both parents and having a mother who knows his sexual orientation. No other variable significantly correlated with parental knowledge of their son's homosexuality.

Regression: Parents' Knowledge of Youth's Sexual Orientation

The tested model, separated according to sex of the youth and parent, proposed parental age, marital status of parents, contact with parents, and satisfaction with parents as independent variables predicting parental knowledge of the youth's sexual orientation. For lesbians this model was significant for mothers and fathers: $F(4, 91) = 2.93, p = .025, r^2 = 11\%$, and $F(4, 88) = 3.20, p = .017, r^2 = 13\%$, respectively. The best mother predictors were a young maternal age, $t(1) = 2.22, p = .03$, and the daughter's report of a satisfying relationship with her, $t(1) = 1.63, p = .11$. The same variables also predicted fathers' knowledge: young paternal age, $t(1) = 2.44, p = .02$, and satisfaction, $t(1) = 1.92, p = .06$. Neither the maternal nor the paternal model significantly predicted male youths' reports of parental knowledge of their homosexuality, $F(4, 183) = .71, p = .588, r^2 = 2\%$, and $F(4, 180) = .99, p = .415, r^2 = 2\%$, respectively.

Table 8.4 Correlations among variables for lesbian youths

Variable	RSE^a	Mother knows	Father knows	Parents married	Mother's age	Father's age	Contact with mother	Contact with father	Satisfaction with mother	Satisfaction with father
RSE										
r	—									
p	.00									
n	97									
Mother knows										
r	.05	—								
p	.61	.00								
n	95	97								
Father knows										
r	-.05	.46	—							
p	.61	.0001	.00							
n	92	93	94							
Parents married										
r	.08	16	-.08	—						
p	.43	.12	.44	.00						
n	96	97	94	98						
Mother's age										
r	-.23	.28	.20	.26	—					
p	.02	.01	.05	.01	.00					
n	94	96	92	96	96					
Father's age										
r	-.18	.23	.25	.25	.84	—				
p	.08	.02	.02	.02	.0001	.00				
n	92	93	94	94	92	94				
Contact with mother										
r	-.12	-.06	-.13	.05	.00	.12	—			
p	.27	.59	.22	.63	.98	.24	.00			
n	95	97	93	97	96	93	97			
Contact with father										
r	-.07	-.11	.14	-.30	-.07	.05	.46	—		
p	.52	.31	.16	.003	.53	.65	.0001	.00		
n	92	93	94	94	92	94	93	94		
Satisfaction with mother										
r	-.26	.19	-.04	.16	.15	.16	.30	-.11	—	
p	.01	.07	.73	.11	.13	.11	.003	.31	.00	
n	95	97	93	97	96	93	97	93	97	
Satisfaction with father										
r	-.16	.01	.25	-.26	.08	.05	.01	.34	.31	—
p	.14	.96	.01	.01	.45	.63	.91	.0001	.003	.00
n	91	92	93	93	91	93	92	93	92	93

^{a}Rosenberg Self-Esteem Scale.

Regression: The Self-Esteem of Youths

Next, the variables age and marital status of the parents, contact and satisfaction with parents, and parents' knowledge of their child's homosexuality were regressed on the youths' self-esteem levels. The mother, but not the father, variables predicted the self-esteem level of lesbians, $F(5, 91) = 3.27, p = .009, r^2 = 15\%$, and $F(5, 88) = 1.06, p = .388, r^2 = 6\%$, respectively. Two individual items were significant contributors: satisfaction with maternal relationship, $t(1) = -2.54, p = .01$, and a young mother, $t(1) = -2.50, p = .01$. Two others approached significance: parents married in the mother model, $t(1) = 1.81, p = .07$, and a young father in the paternal model, $t(1) = -1.79, p = .08$.

Both the mother and the father variables significantly predicted the self-esteem level of the male youths, $F(5, 194) = 4.44$, $p = .0008$, $r^2 = 10\%$, and $F(5, 188) = 3.76$, $p = .003$, $r^2 = 9\%$, respectively. The best individual predictors were satisfaction with mother, $t(1) = -3.54$, $p = .001$, and father, $t(1) = -3.42$, $p = .001$. If the mother knew that her son was gay, his self-esteem was likely to be positive, $t(1) = -2.38$, $p = .02$; this relationship was not the case if the father knew, $t(1) = -.26$, ns. Infrequent contact with the father also predicted high self-esteem for his son, $t(1) = 2.60$, $p = .01$

Table 8.5 Correlations among variables for gay youths

Variable	RSE[a]	Mother knows	Father knows	Parents married	Mother's age	Father's age	Contact with mother	Contact with father	Satisfaction with mother	Satisfaction with father
RSE										
r	—									
p	.00									
n	196									
Mother knows										
r	−.15	—								
p	.03	.00								
n	193	195								
Father knows										
r	−.04	.72	—							
p	.63	.0001	.00							
n	190	188	191							
Parents married										
r	.05	−.03	−.03	—						
p	.52	.68	.64	.00						
n	194	193	190	196						
Mother's age										
r	−.07	.01	−.01	.12	—					
p	.35	.92	.91	.09	.00					
n	189	191	184	189	191					
Father's age										
r	−.08	.02	.04	.14	.87	—				
p	.28	.77	.60	.06	.0001	.00				
n	188	186	187	189	185	189				
Contact with mother										
r	.08	−.06	−.01	−.26	.12	.09	—			
p	.26	.43	.94	.001	.09	.20	.00			
n	193	195	188	193	191	186	195			
Contact with father										
r	.10	.06	.05	−.36	.06	.02	.63	—		
p	.17	.41	.48	.0001	.44	.83	.0001	.00		
n	192	190	190	193	186	189	190	193		
Satisfaction with mother										
r	−.22	.03	−.05	.08	.16	.19	.13	−.01	—	
p	.003	.73	.48	.26	.03	.01	.07	.86	.00	
n	191	193	186	191	190	185	193	188	193	
Satisfaction with father										
r	−.22	−.01	.14	−.12	−.10	−.03	.00	.15	.36	—
p	.002	.85	.06	.11	.20	.71	.96	.04	.0001	.00
n	189	187	187	190	184	187	187	190	187	190

[a]Rosenberg Self-Esteem Scale.

Discussion

General Summary

In the present study, lesbian youths who had positive parental relationships felt comfortable with their sexual orientation and were likely to be out to their parents. Relatively few of the variables tested, however, significantly predicted lesbian self-esteem. Lesbians satisfied with their relationship with their mother and who had young parents were most likely to have a positive self-evaluation. Seemingly unimportant for their self-esteem were parental knowledge and acceptance of their homosexuality, feeling comfortable with their sexual orientation, contact with parents, a satisfying relationship with father, and their parents' marital status.

By contrast, although the parental variables were not related to gay youths' reports of being out to their parents, they served as excellent correlates of their self-esteem level. On the average, if the parents were important for a male's sense of self-worth then their acceptance of his homosexuality predicted his comfortableness with being gay, which in turn significantly predicted his level of self-esteem. In addition, satisfying parental relationships, maternal knowledge of his homosexuality, and having relatively little contact with father predicted positive self-evaluation. Unimportant factors were father's knowledge of son's homosexuality, contact with mother, age of parents, and parents' marital status.

It proved particularly important to consider the sexes separately. A reflected appraisals approach in the context of familial relations "worked" far better for the gay males than it did for the lesbians. This is consistent with previous research on assumed heterosexual samples (Demo et al., 1987) that reported the self-esteem of boys, compared with that of girls, was more strongly related to family relations. Thus, the discriminating power of a reflected appraisals perspective based on family relations is more sensitive to the self-esteem of males than the self-esteem of females for both heterosexual and homosexual youth.

Lesbians who maintained that they had satisfying relationships with their parents and who had relatively young parents were most likely to be out to them. This is consistent with the coming-out-right advice literature. The attempt to replicate these findings with gay youths was unsuccessful. This difference was apparent despite the fact that the lesbians and gay males varied relatively little in their overall responses to the independent variables.

The self-esteem level of the study's participants was highly predictive on the basis of characteristics of the mother for both sexes, but the paternal model was significant only for males. Gay and lesbian youths who reported having satisfying relationships with their mothers had the highest level of self-esteem. In addition, having a young mother was conducive for a positive lesbian self-image, whereas a gay male who was out to his mother and who had a satisfying but infrequent relationship with his father was most likely to report high self-esteem.

State Versus Trait

It is apparent from the data of this study that feeling comfortable with being lesbian or gay is not equivalent to feeling, on a global scale, positive self-evaluation. For sample, adding the variable importance of the parents for one's sense of self-worth, a perception likely to reflect the current state of the relationship, was of far greater significance in predicting a youth's comfortableness with being lesbian or gay than in predicting his or her self-esteem level. The state of feeling comfortable with one's sexual orientation is likely to be more transitory than self-esteem and thus more easily influenced by current perceptions. For example, if one has recently encountered harassment or violence for being homosexual or if one is visiting one's parents in a small, upstate community where religious conservatism reigns and everyone knows the affairs of everyone else, then the uncomfortableness index would probably increase rather dramatically. Self-esteem, on the other hand, as assessed by the Rosenberg Self-Esteem Scale, is considered to be a stable component of one's self-concept or personality, relatively impermeable for most individuals to contextual factors, through the adolescent and adult years (Savin-Williams & Demo, 1984). Although changing physical locations or facing peer rejection may alter one's mood, they are not likely to have an immediate impact on one's assessment of the self as a person of worth and dignity. Thus, the parents' significance in affecting their offspring may depend in part on the permanence of the characteristic under investigation.

Significance of Parents

Results varied depending on whether the perceived attitudes of the mother or those of the father were under consideration. For example, lesbians who felt acceptance from their mother felt comfortable with their sexual orientation, regardless of whether the parents were perceived to be important or not for their sense of self-worth. On the other hand, feeling acceptance from their father predicted their self-esteem level only if they also reported that their parents were important for their sense of self-worth. These trends were not characteristic of the gay males. Thus, separating parental data supplied information that distinguished the attitudes of the male and female youths, highlighting the significance of the mother-daughter relationship for the average lesbian's sense of comfortableness with her sexual identity. This bond is even more apparent in regard to the daughter's self-evaluation: The lesbians' self-esteem scores were related to feelings of satisfaction with mother but not with father. The mother was also important for gay male youths' level of self-esteem. The maternal variables were more highly predictive of the acceptance → comfortableness → self-esteem sequence than were the variables in the paternal model. Male youths who were out to their mother had high levels of self-esteem, whereas with fathers infrequent contact predicted positive self-esteem.

Perhaps the significance of the mother lies in her unique role as "mother" and the seemingly more distant and less satisfying relationship that many gay males and lesbians have with their father. This finding is congruent with other studies (reviewed by Bell, Weinberg, & Hammersmith, 1981a). These mother–father differences do not, however, warrant support for the traditional "dominant mother/aloof father" syndrome proposed as a causative factor in the development of homosexuality by psychoanalytic writers, primarily because similar relationships also characterize heterosexual youth. Rather, a more parsimonious explanation is that for many adolescents in our society, regardless of sexual orientation, mothers are viewed as considerably more supportive, warm, and emotional than are fathers. Apparently, this support is most likely to come from young mothers when the issue is their daughter's sexual identity. Lesbians in this study who had a young mother were most likely to be out to their mother and to have positive self-esteem.

Gay males reported highest levels of satisfaction with young mothers. As suggested by the coming-out-right literature, the significance of the mother's youthfulness may reside in her own child-rearing culture that encouraged her to be open and tolerant, if not accepting, of homosexuality. This question requires further study.

Reflected Appraisals Model

A reflected appraisals perspective with parents posed as significant others received mixed support, with several important limitations and refinements. In terms of support, congruent with the reflected appraisals prediction, lesbians felt most comfortable with their sexual orientation if they also reported that their mother and father accepted (or would accept if they knew) their sexual orientation. Adding the variable importance of the parents to self-worth increased this relationship with father acceptance (as predicted) but not with mother acceptance. As noted earlier, lesbians in the current study were comfortable with their sexual orientation if they felt acceptance by their mother, regardless of how important they reported that their parents were for their sense of self-worth. Also, in terms of limitations, the reflected appraisals model was not particularly helpful in predicting lesbians' self-esteem level. Adding importance of the parents to self-worth changed little for the mother acceptance → comfortableness → self-esteem model; the father acceptance model now approached significance.

The reflected appraisals perspective received stronger support when data from the gay males were considered. Feeling acceptance from mother or father predicted those who felt most at ease with their sexual orientation only if the parents were perceived as important components of their sense of self-worth. This finding affirms Rosenberg's (1979) injunction that one must document the significance of supposedly "significant others" for one's self-evaluation. Furthermore, the reflected appraisals model significantly predicted self-esteem level among gay males: Those who were most comfortable with their sexual orientation had the highest level of self-esteem.

It is important to recognize as well that reflected appraisals added relatively little to our understanding of effective and evaluative components of lesbian and gay lives. The significant results accounted for relatively little (9 to 15% at best) of the variance in feeling comfortable with one's sexual orientation, coming out to parents, and one's self-esteem level. Apparently, there are critical factors other than reported current relationships with parents that are responsible for these variables (see Chapters 6 and 7). Parents are not usually perceived as the first line of support; same-age friends or older gay men and lesbians usually assume this role (Sandfort, 1983; Straver, 1976).

This does not necessarily imply that the family is unimportant in these matters. Early parent–infant interactions, physical affection, childhood rearing practices, and family religious teachings may be far better predictors of the state of comfortableness with one's sexual orientation, the expression of that to others, and a global sense of self-evaluation. At this point, we simply do not know. Thus, the results from this investigation provide only a small piece of the answer in these highly important spheres.

Because data collection was cross-sectional and not longitudinal, issues of prediction are tenuous at best. Positive self-esteem might just as easily "cause" one to come out as the reverse assumption of the tested model (that coming-out status predicts self-esteem level). For example, it is not clear (a) whether a satisfying parental relationship encourages a lesbian to come out to her parents or the relationship is satisfying because the lesbian youth has come out to them, and (b) whether satisfaction with parents causes a gay male's high self-esteem or is the result of it. The coming-out-right advice literature was not particularly helpful in sorting these relationships out because it suggested that both are true.

Because the theoretical and empirical coming-out literature largely ignores the role of the parents for the adolescent, it sheds relatively little light in proposing and testing various causal pathways. The present research provides data that are especially pertinent in documenting the relationships among parental characteristics, the coming-out process, and self-esteem.

9

Gender Variations

OVERVIEW

The sexes were compared on all study variables in terms of how frequently they described the youths. Age trends were also noted in these gender variations. The perspective assumed was that when gender variations were explored, behavioral and verbal expressions of differences would generally be more quantitative than qualitative. This view has been expressed previously: "Differences between males and females reside in differential frequencies of exhibition of behavior rather than in whether or not a particular behavior is expressed" (Reinisch & Sanders, 1984, p. 409). According to this orthogonal model, individuals have the capacity for expressing various behaviors that are, at a group level, more characteristic of one sex than the other. Individuals vary immensely in their capacity and willingness to behave like their respective sex—as a result of unique combinations of biological, psychological, and cultural reasons. Thus, when individuals are grouped according to sex, mean group differences will be apparent, but within-group variations will also be excessive.

It is no secret, nor should it be surprising, that research on homosexuality reflects the prevalent male bias of the social sciences. Early research was based primarily on samples of homosexual men. The male preponderance is less marked today, but characteristic of the literature nevertheless. The reasons for the male bias are far too numerous and complex to detail here, but they include the greater visibility of gay men, a male-centered ideological perspective of researchers, a greater number of men in professional and other research positions, and the desexualized view of female relationships. In the 1980s research has taken the lesbian experience more seriously (e.g., Bell & Weinberg, 1978; Ettorre, 1980; Kehoe, 1986; Krieger, 1982; Ponse, 1980; Richardson, 1981a; Sang, 1978).

As a result, the relative weight of sex and sexual orientation has become both a theoretical and an empirical consideration. From earliest experiences of life, the worlds of pre-gay and pre-lesbian youth are qualitatively divergent from their straight peers. It is unclear, however, if the common perceptions, cognitions, and experiences that they share because of their sexual orientation are more similar than the perspectives that they share with heterosexual members of their sex. G. Sanders (1980) assumed the latter:

> Owing to these sex-role stereotyped patterns of upbringing and socialization, men and women develop separately and shape their lives differently. Seen in this context, hetero- and homosexual women are first and foremost women, and hetero- and homosexual men are first and foremost men. (p. 306)

This issue, however, has seldom been addressed empirically because samples of lesbians, gay males, heterosexual females, and heterosexual males are rarely included in the same study.

The one aspect of this debate that could be addressed with the present research was the degree of similarity among the gay and lesbian youths. Each of the seven clusters of variables used throughout this study—sociodemographics, attitudes and interests, gay-related activities and attitudes, support of family and friends, love affairs, self-descriptions, and self-worth—was addressed, first in frequency of response and second as related to predicting self-esteem level. Although the age spread in the current sample was relatively narrow and there were few youths in the youngest age groups, it is instructive for future research endeavors to consider gender variations from the perspective of age. The sample was divided into roughly three equal age groups: 14 to 19, 20 to 21, and 22 to 23 years of age.

DESCRIPTIVE DATA

Sociodemographic Variables

There were no significant differences between the male and female youths on age, education, ed-age, community size raised in, report of pubertal onset, and parents' occupational status. There was a slight tendency within the youngest age grouping, the 14- to 19-year-olds, for males to be slightly younger and less educated.[1] This reflects the absence of 14- to 15-year-old lesbians in the sample.

The lack of difference found in age of pubertal onset is counter to the well-documented finding that females mature physically 1 to 2 years earlier than males (Nottelmann et al., 1987). The females' report of a mean of 11.87 years is clearly a late age for pubertal onset, whereas the males' mean of 11.95 years is similar to other reports of males in the literature. One possible explanation is that the lesbians were as a group late maturers, but there is little theoretical or empirical support for this conclusion. More likely, the late onset of maturation could be construed not as a physical quirk in this sample but the result of lesbians using later developmental markers to assess pubertal onset than males. If the males were identifying early developments such as pubic hair or genitalia growth as pubertal onset, then their average age of pubertal onset is reasonable; if the females were using a later pubertal event, such as menarche, as pubertal onset, then the failure to find a sex difference in pubertal timing is understandable. Specifying the particulars for each sex in assessing pubertal onset would have prevented this interpretation dilemma.

Unless the males were recalling a late event, such as the growth spurt, the present data add little support to those (Storms, 1980; Sullivan, 1953; Tripp, 1975) who proposed that males who are early maturers are most likely to be gay. I am currently conducting a follow-up study with late adolescent gay males and one question asked is for age and event of pubertal onset. For the vast majority of the 34 interviewed, pubertal onset clearly means pubic hair onset. I do not have comparable data for the lesbians.

---

[1]For age ($N = 28, 69$), $t(1) = 1.91, p = .06$; for education ($N = 28, 69$), $t(1) = 2.31, p = .024$. In the analyses and text, age differences in the gender relationships are presented to assist the examination of age variations in gender patterns by future investigators with larger sample sizes than the present sample. Little is made of these findings in this report because of the large error factor in the analyses. N represents the number of 14- to 19-year-old females and males, respectively, that were compared.

Thus, at least on the level of sociodemographic characteristics the gay and lesbian samples appeared to be quite similar. On other dimensions, however, the two diverged.

Attitudes and Interests

In Chapter 5 it was noted that relatively little research has explored the attitudes and interests variables included in this study. As is the case with other variables examined in the present study, the Bell and Weinberg study (1978) is the notable exception.[2] Among gay and lesbian adults in the Bell and Weinberg study, females were more likely than males to consider themselves Democrats (47% vs. 36%) rather than Republicans (10% vs. 17%) and somewhat less likely to describe their political orientation as conservative (3% vs. 8%). Ferguson and Finkler (1978) noted that most (66%) lesbians in their sample claimed to be feminists. In their attitudes toward men and women, each sex considered same-sex individuals to be psychologically superior to members of the other sex (Bell & Weinberg, 1978). Lesbians and gay males were equally not religious (81% and 79%, respectively) and seldom attended a religious service (87% and 82%, respectively). Counter to these findings, Chicago gay men were more mainstream religious while lesbians were more likely to report personalized religious belief (McKirnan & Peterson, 1986). Gay males were more likely than lesbians to never attend sporting events (69% vs. 56%) or participate in a sports activity (62% vs. 69%) during the last 12 months (Bell & Weinberg, 1978). In grade school, 20% of the females said they felt different because of an interest in sports, and 48% of the males said they felt different because they did not like sports (Bell, Weinberg, & Hammersmith, 1981b).

In the present sample, lesbians and gay males differed sharply on particular attitudes and interests (Table 9.1). The lesbians were considerably more politically liberal and stronger supporters of feminism. Interest in and skill at athletics were significantly greater among the lesbians. Gay males, on the other hand, reported a greater degree of religiosity.

The gender differences in feminism and sports interests were highly significant for all age groups, whereas the political and religiosity differences were significant only among the 20- to 21-year-old group.

Thus, the lesbian youths differed from gay males in ways similar to Bell and Weinberg's adult population. They were more politically liberal, more interested and involved in sports, and less religiously inclined. The latter is somewhat of a novel finding. These differences are certainly not true gender differences because they are inconsistent with general gender patterns in the larger population. For example, males are generally more sports oriented, and females more religious. The data presented here cannot explain these differences between gay and lesbian youths. My best guess is that they are indicative of the radicalization of lesbians (double minority status) and the gender-atypical behavioral and sex role characteristics of lesbians and gay males.

[2]In all references to Bell and Weinberg (1978) in this chapter, the comparison is with their findings on White and not Black adults, primarily because the present sample was essentially a White one.

Table 9.1 Significant differences between gay males and lesbians in attitudes and interests across and within ages

Variable	Ns		t	p
	Females	Males		
Across ages				
Political outlook	103	211	4.34	.0001
Feminism	101	211	5.87	.0001
Religiosity	101	210	1.92	.056
Sports	103	214	5.16	.0001
Within ages[a]				
Political outlook				
20–21	52	86	5.11	.0001
Feminism				
14–19	27	68	3.60	.0006
20–21	51	86	3.77	.0003
22–23	23	57	2.73	.008
Religiosity				
20–21	51	87	2.80	.006
Sports				
14–19	28	69	3.43	.001
20–21	52	87	2.89	.005
22–23	23	58	3.00	.005

[a]Ages are in years.

Gay-Related Activities and Attitudes

As was noted in Chapter 3, a nearly universal finding in empirical research is that males recognize their homosexuality and come out at an earlier age than do females (Miranda, 1986; G. Sanders, 1980; Schafer, 1977; Van Wyk & Geist, 1984). In the Netherlands (G. Sanders, 1980), boys discovered their same-sex attraction at age 13 years; girls, at 16 years. Full awareness occurred at ages 15 and 18 years, respectively. Ages differ among the studies: 14.9 years for males and 18.2 years for females for first having "suspicions" in a West German population (Schafer, 1977); 12.0 years for males and 13.9 years for females for first learning about homosexuality in a reanalysis of Kinsey's data (Van Wyk & Geist, 1984); and 11.6 years for males and 16.5 years of age for females for first time sexually aroused by same-sex stimuli in a large-scale U.S. sample (Bell et al., 1981b). Across several cultures and time periods, as a group males recognized their homosexuality at an earlier age.

Another common finding in the literature is that males report a larger number of sexual partners but females are more likely to have had heterosexual experiences, especially during adolescence. In regard to number of sex partners, Bell and Weinberg (1978) reported that 75% of their gay sample had had 100 or more sexual partners in their lifetime, whereas 2% of the lesbians had had that many. Others supported this finding. Saghir, Robins, and Walbran (1969) found that 94% of the males but only 15% of the females had had more than 15 sexual partners; in Loney's (1972) study, the males averaged 19.4 homosexual partners, and the females 3.7 partners. These results are also characteristic of West German gay men and lesbians: The average number of homosexual sex partners was 75 for males and 7 for females, and the percentages of those with more than 50 partners were

56% of males and 5% of females (Schafer, 1977). In Chicago, 6% of the lesbians and 19% of the gay men had two or more new sex partners per month (McKirnan & Peterson, 1986).

Lesbians are generally more involved in heterosexual activities. Comparing the two sexes on a number of heterosexual experiences, Bell and Weinberg (1978) reported greater frequency among females than males in heterosexual coitus (83% vs. 64%), receiving (70% vs. 40%) and giving (71% vs. 35%) masturbation, and sex dreams (55% vs. 33%). There were few differences in guilt feelings with either homosexual or heterosexual sex. The lesbians in Loney's (1972) sample averaged 5.3 and the males 1.3 heterosexual partners. Before the age of 20 years, 70% of the females and 49% of the males in another study felt heterosexual arousal (Saghir et al., 1969). Lesbians were more likely to heterosexually date (79% vs. 48%) as adolescents and young adults and to have more heterosexual partners (31% had four or more; males, 17%). This was also true among West Germans (Schafer, 1977): 38% of the lesbians and 20% of the gay males had had a heterosexual contact during the previous 12 months, and 56% of the females but only 19% of the males had had heterosexual before homosexual encounters. In all studies reviewed females were more likely than males to heterosexually marry, for example, 14% versus 6% (Schafer, 1977) and 35% versus 20% (Bell & Weinberg, 1978). Schafer (1977) noted, "Lesbian women label their homosexual needs at a later age and thus inevitably remain 'fellow travelers' in the typical heterosexual process of socialization—dating, kissing, going steady, intercourse—for a larger period of time than do homosexual men" (p. 358).

Males are generally more likely than females to describe themselves as exclusively or predominantly homosexual. In the Bell and Weinberg (1978) study, 92% (behavior) and 86% (feelings) of the males rated themselves on the Kinsey scale as a 5 or 6; the comparable female percentages were 87% and 78%. This gender difference was similarly reported by adults recalling their childhood and adolescence: predominantly homosexual in behavior (56% of males and 22% of females) and feelings (59% of males and 44% of females) (Bell et al., 1981a). Kirkpatrick and Morgan (1980) offered the following interpretation of this trend for females to report a higher incidence of bisexuality and for males to report exclusive homosexuality:

> In women, homosexuality and heterosexuality do not appear to be at opposite ends of a continuum as Kinsey et al. (1953) suggested they were. Rather, the two trends might be seen as running a parallel course, capable of intermingling and of changing positions of ascendancy in consciousness and behavior under certain circumstances. (p. 360)

Although males in the Bell et al. study (1981a) reported an earlier age of feeling gay and a more marked exclusivity to homosexuality, females generally had fewer problems with their sexual orientation. They were less likely than males (58% vs. 64%) to describe their childhood and adolescence in negative terms and as adults to have no regret for being homosexual (64% vs. 49%). However, they were more likely to have considered giving up their homosexual activity (38% vs. 29%) (Bell & Weinberg, 1978). Similar results were found in other samples of adults. In an early, ground-breaking study one-half of the females but two-thirds of the males desired to change their sexual orientation during their adolescence and young adulthood (Saghir & Robins, 1973). As adults the lesbians were less concerned than gay males with their physical attractiveness, staying young, and the social and economic effects of their homosexuality. Saghir and Robins (1980) concluded that being a lesbian entailed less conflict and internal turmoil than being a gay man. G. Sanders (1980) reached the same conclusion in his Netherlands sample:

> *The girls display to a considerably more limited degree than do the boys feelings of personal insecurity, social isolation, and of feeling socially threatened as a result of acknowledging a connection between the nature of their own feelings and the label "homosexual". (p. 303)*

Congruent with this, 91% of Loney's (1972) lesbian sample but only 55% of the males was satisfied with their sexual adjustment. The sexes were equal, however, on desire to change sexual orientation (35% of the females and 36% of the males).

Bell and Weinberg (1978) reported that males and females were equally likely to join a homophile organization (24% of males and 21% of females), to attend a meeting at least once a week (29% of males and 31% of females), and in general to be highly involved in political organizations (39% of males and 37% of females). Males were more likely to go to a gay bar at least once a week (49% vs. 28%). In the Netherlands, gay males participated more in the "homosexual scene" (G. Sanders, 1980).

In terms of these variables, the gay males in the present study should have been more inclined than the lesbians to report being exclusively homosexual, having felt gay at an earlier age, having had many homosexual partners but few heterosexual partners, and feeling that their sexual orientation is beyond their control. The lesbians were expected to be more satisfied (comfortableness) with their homosexuality. All of these relationships were confirmed at a significant level (Table 9.2). As one might expect, lesbians reported more sexual contact with other females; gay males, with males. The overall number of sexual contacts averaged only somewhat higher among the males, nine versus six for females. The lesbians, on the other hand, averaged more heterosexual sexual partners, four versus the gay males' mean of one.

There were no gender differences in involvement with lesbian and gay rights organizations, socializing with other lesbians and gays, participation in lesbian and gay activities, or attending lesbian or gay bars. All but the last finding are consistent with the literature. Males were also more likely to read homosexually related periodicals.

Most of these relationships were true across the age groups. Two exceptions emerged: Only among the 20- to 21-year-olds were the males more likely to report being exclusively gay and to read a greater number of periodicals.

Thus, in most respects the gender differences in the current sample of lesbian and gay youths mirror findings from studies with lesbian and gay adults. At a youthful age, the gay males were more likely than the lesbians to recognize their inevitable "commitment" to homosexuality; the lesbian youths, similar to older lesbians, felt more comfortable with their homosexuality than did males—perhaps in part because lesbians are more likely to believe that they are homosexual by choice (e.g., Ferguson & Finkler, 1978) and to feel that they are less exclusively homosexual. Perhaps satisfaction resides more strongly under conditions of choice than of fate. The cause–effect cycle is difficult to break when considering these issues. For example, perhaps lesbians feel they can choose to be homosexual or bisexual because they are more satisfied with their sexual orientation.

The gay youths in the present sample were far less likely than their older male peers to be involved in homosexual sex and to attend a gay bar. How much of this

Table 9.2 Significant differences between gay males and lesbians in
gay-related activites and attitudes across and within ages

Variable	Ns		*t*	*p*
	Females	Males		
Across ages				
Sexual orientation	101	213	3.74	.0003
Age first felt homosexual	101	208	5.22	.0001
Beyond control	101	204	6.46	.0001
Give up desire	100	207	2.99	.003
Sex partners				
Number female	103	213	6.15	.0001
Number male	102	212	8.01	.0001
Periodicals	103	213	3.05	.003
Within ages[a]				
Sexual orientation				
20–21	50	86	3.48	.0009
Age first felt homosexual				
14–19	27	67	3.39	.001
20–21	51	85	3.53	.0007
22–23	23	56	2.34	.03
Beyond control				
14–19	27	64	3.16	.003
20–21	51	83	4.83	.0001
22–23	23	57	2.92	.006
Give up desire				
14–19	27	64	2.34	.03
22–23	23	58	2.01	.05
Sex partners				
Number female				
14–19	28	68	2.98	.005
20–21	52	87	4.78	.0001
22–23	23	58	3.24	.003
Number male				
14–19	28	65	4.05	.0002
20–21	51	86	5.30	.0001
22–23	23	58	5.02	.0001
Periodicals				
20–21	52	86	2.14	.03

[a]Ages are in years.

difference is an age rather than a cohort effect is not possible to determine. Data
were collected before AIDS consciousness emerged and before many states
changed their drinking age. The failure to find a gender difference in bar attendance may be due to the college-oriented nature of the sample (frequent bar attendance for either sex usually parallels academic failure) or to the fact that the local
Ithaca, New York, bar is equally inviting to lesbians and gay males. The sexes also
appeared similarly social in all other respects.

Support of Family and Friends

Knowledge distinguishing between the friendship patterns of lesbians and gay
males is considerably limited. Bell and Weinberg (1978) reported few gender differences in the number of "good, close friends": 2% of each sex replied having

none and 41% said they had six or more. Lesbians were slightly more likely to have cross-sex and heterosexual friends; 15% of the females but 29% of the males said they had only same-sex friends. One-quarter of the lesbians' same-sex friends were homosexual; the percentage for the gay males was nearly twice (44%) that level. Males were also more likely than females (40% vs. 29%) to report relatively high contact with friends. These trends were apparent during childhood and adolescence (Bell et al., 1981a).

Relationships with parents during childhood and adolescence were somewhat dependent on the sex of the parent (Bell et al., 1981a, 1981b). Lesbians were more likely to describe having a positive relationship with their fathers than were gay males (32% vs. 22%). Although relationships with mother were considerably more positive in general than for fathers, gay males reported having more positive feelings toward their mothers than did lesbians (65% vs. 39%). Sibling relations did not vary between the sexes. For example, both lesbians (60%) and gay males (54%) felt close to a sister while growing up.

Only two significant findings distinguished the lesbians from the gay males in the present sample across all three age groups: Lesbians reported having more lesbian friends and gay males reported having more gay friends (Table 9.3). Lesbians reported feeling more acceptance from their closest academic advisor at ages 14 to 19 years and 22 to 23 years; males, from their mother at ages 20 to 21 years. At this same age, gay males reported having more heterosexual male friends than did the lesbians. There were no significant gender differences at any age for perceived acceptance of father, sibling, and best heterosexual female or male friend or for the reported number of bisexual and heterosexual female friends.

Gender differences in friendship patterns and in feelings of acceptance from

Table 9.3 Significant differences between gay males and lesbians in support of family and friends across and within ages

Variable	Ns		t	p
	Females	Males		
Across ages				
Lesbian friends	94	195	7.53	.0001
Gay friends	93	202	4.59	.0001
Within ages[a]				
Lesbian friends				
14–19	25	63	3.32	.002
20–21	48	80	5.78	.0001
22–23	21	52	3.67	.0007
Gay friends				
14–19	23	65	3.62	.0006
20–21	50	81	2.93	.004
22–23	20	56	2.64	.01
Professor				
14–19	19	37	2.52	.01
22–23	19	37	2.39	.02
Mother				
20–21	51	85	2.46	.02
Heterosexual male friends				
20–21	47	80	2.18	.03

[a]Ages are in years.

family and friends were essentially nonexistent among the sampled youths. Each reported having more same-sex, same-sexual-orientation friends, but these findings are hardly revelatory. The incongruity between the results of Bell and Weinberg (1978) and the present study may reflect (a) a changing pattern in which gay males are recognizing the importance of social support (more similar to females than to heterosexual males), (b) an age difference associated with the need for support in developing identity consolidation during adolescence, and/or (c) a by-product of variations, aside from age, within the populations sampled. It appears, however, from these findings and the self-description and sense of self-worth results reported below that the sexes in the sample cannot be easily distinguished on the importance they place on close, intimate relationships with others.

Love Affairs

A consistent finding across several studies is that lesbians are more likely than gay males to be in a current love relationship, to experience love affairs, and to maintain such affairs for a lengthy period of time. Loney (1972) reported 82% of the females but only 22% of the males had been in a "same-sex marriage" prior to data collection. For Saghir et al. (1969), the percentages were 93% of females and 61% of males; and for Schafer (1977), 72% of females and 59% of males. In the Schafer study, 43% of the male "steady relationships" lasted less than 6 months (vs. 29% among lesbians) and 21% for more than 2 years (vs. 27% among lesbians). Lesbians also viewed relationships as more serious than did the gay men; they more highly valued living together, taking vacations together, and demanding sexual fidelity. One-half of the gay men with a steady partner had had sex with more than 10 men during the last year. Among Chicago gay men and women (McKirnan & Peterson, 1986), males were more likely than lesbians to be single (53% vs. 32%); lesbians, to value monogamous relationships and to have fewer sex partners.

Bell and Weinberg (1978) reported 40% of their lesbians and 24% of their gay males had had five or more relationships. Although gay males had experienced homosexual sex several years before lesbians (Bell et al., 1981a; Saghir et al., 1969; Schafer, 1977), lesbians began relationships earlier—40% before age 19 years, compared with 31% for gay males (Bell & Weinberg, 1978). Lesbians were more likely to live with their first partner (65% vs. 52%); to be in love with her (90% vs. 78%); to stay in the relationship longer (4 or more years: 31% vs. 22%); and to feel that they received from the relationship self-insight (35% vs. 26%) and self-confidence (24% vs. 13%). More lesbians were in a relationship at data collection time (72% vs. 51%) and felt "coupled" with the partner (67% vs. 56%). The males, however, were more likely to have been in their current affair longer— 43% versus the lesbians' 31% for 4 or more years.

Results from the current study essentially affirmed these gender differences. Across all age groups and for the sample as a whole, lesbians reported more love relationships, were more likely to be in a current relationship, and had more relationships that lasted a long time, especially at ages 20 to 21 years (Table 9.4). For the youngest age group, the first relationship was more likely to have been with a member of the same sex for lesbians than for gay males; for the oldest age

Table 9.4 Significant differences between gay males and lesbians in
          love affairs across and within ages

	Ns			
Variable	Females	Males	t	p
Across ages				
Number of love affairs	99	208	4.94	.0001
Current affair	98	204	4.19	.0001
Longevity	89	141	1.94	.05
Within ages[a]				
Number of love affairs				
14–19	26	69	2.85	.007
20–21	51	83	2.62	.01
22–23	22	56	3.13	.004
Current affair				
14–19	26	66	2.17	.04
20–21	50	81	2.86	.005
22–23	22	57	2.00	.05
Longevity				
20–21	46	59	1.89	.06
Sex of first lover				
14–19	19	27	2.21	.03
Age of first affair				
22–23	19	32	2.41	.02

[a]Ages are in years.

group, lesbians reported a younger age of first relationship. The two sexes were equally likely to engage in a large percentage of homosexual relationships.

These findings lend further support to the view that females are better able than males to initiate and sustain love relationships, a view that is frequently cited as evidence for the importance of femaleness and maleness in understanding lesbian and gay development. For example, Tripp (1975) noted that short-term sexual affairs and promiscuous contacts are "mainly the province of men and not women." This sex difference is more clouded in heterosexual relationships because of the restraints women place on men to be faithful. "But in homosexuality, the difference between the sexes is sharply drawn, not only by the ease of male–male contacts but by the near-total lack of promiscuity among lesbians" (p. 154). The female's desire for supportive and intimate relationships will thus engender longer and more frequent love affairs than is found among males. The lesson of lesbianism supports "the ancient idea that women generally supply much more of the glue and the constancy of ordinary marriages than men do" (p. 164). Thus, the argument concludes, in homosexual relations the true nature of male and female patterns emerge. This matter is pursued in a later section of this chapter.

Self-Descriptions and Self-Worth

Relatively few studies have compared gay males and lesbians on personality characteristics. In one study, gay males were more hypersensitive and less competitive than were lesbians (Saghir & Robins, 1973). Siegelman (1972a, 1972b) studied 307 gay males (mean age = 36 years) and 84 lesbians (mean age = 30 years) who were middle to upper middle class in social status. Both samples were recruited from homophile organizations, bookstore advertisements, and friends. Comparing scores on various adjustment measures revealed few gender differences on the characteristics tender minded, submissive, trusting, dependency, and nurturance. Lesbians were considerably more depressed and goal directed; gay males, more anxious. Males were slightly more alienated and neurotic. In another study (Bell & Weinberg, 1978), gay males felt greater tension but there was no gender difference on depression.

Of the 17 self-descriptions in the present study, only 3 distinguished males from females: Gay males more frequently described themselves as having a muscular build, and lesbians more frequently described themselves as athletic and understanding of others (Table 9.5). These differences and others were more specific to particular age groupings. More so than female youths, male youths described themselves as accomplished in a chosen field at the youngest age and as aggressive at ages 20 to 21 years. Lesbians were more likely to characterize themselves as athletic at ages 14 to 21 years. On the vast majority of self-descriptors there were relatively few gender differences.

Examination of variables that are important for one's self-worth reveals that lesbians and gay males differed on only several items (Table 9.6). The lesbians more frequently reported that having close female friends was important to them; the gay males reported that having close male friends, physical looks, and material possessions and religion were important to them.

The close female friends difference was consistent across all age groups and the close male friends was characteristic for all but the oldest age group. Having possessions was a significant gender distinguisher, with males higher at ages 14 to

Table 9.5 Significant differences between gay males and lesbians in self-descriptions across and within ages

| | Ns | | | |
Variable	Females	Males	t	p
Across ages				
Muscular	102	212	2.07	.04
Athletic	103	213	4.47	.0001
Understanding	103	213	1.97	.05
Within ages[a]				
Accomplished				
14–19	25	65	2.10	.04
Aggressive				
20–21	52	85	3.21	.002
Athletic				
14–19	28	69	3.09	.003
20–21	52	86	3.14	.002

[a]Ages are in years.

Table 9.6 Significant differences between gay males and lesbians in
sense of self-worth across and within ages

Variable	Ns		t	p
	Females	Males		
Across ages				
Female friends	103	212	9.78	.0001
Male friends	103	212	6.17	.0001
Physical looks	102	213	2.36	.02
Possessions	103	213	3.95	.0001
Religion	103	213	1.98	.05
Within ages[a]				
Female friends				
14–19	28	68	4.46	.0001
20–21	52	87	6.56	.0001
22–23	23	57	5.63	.0001
Male friends				
14–19	28	68	3.87	.0004
20–21	52	87	4.88	.0001
Physical looks				
20–21	51	86	2.22	.03
Possessions				
14–19	28	69	3.34	.0002
22–23	23	58	2.47	.02
Religion				
20–21	52	87	2.18	.03
Relationship with parents				
22–23	23	58	2.29	.03

[a]Ages are in years.

19 and 22 to 23 years. At ages 20 to 21 years physical looks and religion were
significantly higher for males, and at ages 22 to 23 years lesbians were more likely
to list parents as an important element in their sense of self-worth.

Distinguishing between males and females on personality characteristics and
self-worth qualities has been a rarity in research on homosexuality, and perhaps for
good reason. Unlike studies with heterosexual samples, very few gender differences emerged in the present analysis. Those that did were, more so than with
other variables investigated, age bound. Males were slightly more in tune than
lesbian youths to materialism, describing themselves as having muscular build and
reporting that physical looks and material possessions were important for their
sense of self-worth. On the other hand, they also more frequently attributed religion to their sense of self-worth. Patterns are difficult to interpret.

Age Trends Across Variables

There were relatively few systematic differences among the gay males or lesbians as a function of age when they were divided into three age groups: 14- to 19-
year-olds, 20- to 21-year-olds, and 22- to 23-year-olds. Among the oldest male
youths the first love affair, homosexual or heterosexual, began at a late age and,
compared with younger gay males, there was an increased perception that one was
out to a best heterosexual male friend (Table 9.7). Only two age trends were

Table 9.7 Age patterns for males and females across select study
variables

Variable/age group[a]	Ns		t	p
	Males			
Age of first affair				
14–19 vs. 20–21	27	49	1.40	.17
20–21 vs. 22–23	49	32	1.89	.06
14–19 vs. 22–23	27	32	3.27	.002
Out to male friends				
14–19 vs. 20–21	65	75	1.59	.11
20–21 vs. 22–23	75	49	1.63	.11
14–19 vs. 22–23	65	49	3.03	.003
	Females			
Accomplished				
16–19 vs. 20–21	25	48	1.69	.10
20–21 vs. 22–23	48	23	2.10	.04
16–19 vs. 22–23	25	23	3.04	.004
Affair longevity				
16–19 vs. 20–21	22	46	1.44	.16
20–21 vs. 22–23	46	21	1.72	.10
16–19 vs. 22–23	22	21	2.26	.03

[a]Ages are in years.

consistent in the lesbian sample. With increasing age, lesbians were more likely to describe themselves as "accomplished" and to report that their love affairs lasted a long time. These findings indicate that with age there is an increased tendency for being out (males), feeling self-mastery (females), and having love relationships that have survived (females) or have been delayed to a later age (males). The uniqueness of each of the three age divisions is considered below.

Males

The 14- to 19-year-old males were clearly the most unique of any of the six sex/age groups. Compared with their older male peers, they were less likely to be out to others, especially to mother, closest sibling, and best heterosexual female friend, and less likely to feel that their homosexuality was accepted by their mother, father, best female friend, and best male friend. As might be expected, young gay males reported the fewest number of homosexual sexual experiences and love relationships. Material possessions were extremely important for their sense of self-worth, and they were unlikely to describe themselves as aggressive (Table 9.8).

The 20- to 21-year-old gay males were frequent gay bar patrons; they also felt acceptance by their academic advisor/professor. The oldest gay youths, the 22- to 23-year-olds, reported having the largest number of female sex partners; on the other hand, their gay love relationships were likely to last a long period of time. They were the least concerned with physical appearance.

Females

Somewhat surprisingly, the 16- to 19-year-old lesbians were most likely to report being out to mother (Table 9.9). Lesbians 20 to 21 years of age were the

Table 9.8 Significant and near-significant unique variations for each
age group among males

Variable/age group	Ns		t	p
14- to 19-year-olds				
Out to mother				
vs. 20–21	67	85	1.73	.09
vs. 22–23	67	57	2.14	.03
Out to sibling				
vs. 20–21	67	81	1.76	.08
vs. 22–23	67	54	1.87	.06
Out to female friend				
vs. 20–21	65	83	2.14	.03
vs. 22–23	65	54	2.48	.01
Mother accepts				
vs. 20–21	65	85	2.18	.03
vs. 22–23	65	57	1.36	.18
Father accepts				
vs. 20–21	59	85	1.30	.20
vs. 22–23	59	56	1.82	.07
Female friend accepts				
vs. 20–21	63	83	2.44	.02
vs. 22–23	63	54	2.38	.02
Male friend accepts				
vs. 20–21	63	75	2.13	.04
vs. 22–23	63	49	2.36	.02
Male partners				
vs. 20–21	68	86	2.23	.03
vs. 22–23	68	58	2.90	.004
Number of love affairs				
vs. 20–21	69	83	1.92	.06
vs. 22–23	69	56	1.82	.07
Possessions				
vs. 20–21	68	87	2.22	.03
vs. 22–23	68	58	1.94	.05
Aggressive				
vs. 20–21	69	85	2.22	.03
vs. 22–23	69	56	2.20	.03
20- to 21-year-olds				
Bar attendance				
vs. 14–19	87	69	2.67	.009
vs. 22–23	87	58	1.76	.08
Professor accepts				
vs. 14–19	62	37	2.19	.03
vs. 22–23	62	37	1.89	.06
22- to 23-year-olds				
Female partners				
vs. 14–19	58	68	2.73	.007
vs. 20–21	58	87	2.48	.02
Physical looks				
vs. 14–19	58	69	1.78	.08
vs. 20–21	58	86	1.79	.08
Affair longevity				
vs. 14–19	42	40	1.72	.09
vs. 20–21	42	59	1.81	.07

Note. Second number under *N*s represents the comparison group.
Ages are in years.

Table 9.9 Significant and near-significant unique variations for each
           age group among females

Variable/age group	Ns		t	p
16- to 19-year-olds				
Out to mother				
vs. 20–21	28	51	2.23	.03
vs. 22–23	28	21	2.81	.007
20- to 21-year-olds				
Liberal				
vs. 16–19	52	28	2.16	.04
vs. 22–23	52	23	2.39	.02
Professor accepts				
vs. 16–19	37	19	1.82	.07
vs. 22–23	37	19	1.98	.05
22- to 23-year-olds				
Female partners				
vs. 16–19	23	28	2.49	.02
vs. 20–21	23	52	2.13	.04
Love affairs				
vs. 16–19	22	26	1.93	.06
vs. 20–21	22	51	1.53	.13

Note. Second number under *N*s represents the comparison group.
Ages are in years.

most liberal in political beliefs but, in contrast to the same-age gay males, felt little acceptance from their academic advisor. The oldest lesbians reported having the largest number of female sex partners and love affairs.

DISCUSSION

The question raised by Kirkpatrick and Morgan (1980, p. 357) concerning female homosexuality—whether it is a mirror image of male homosexuality or a specifically female sexual style—has been answered by most writers in a fairly uniform chord: It is more female than homosexual. On the basis of their experiences in a clinical practice, Kirkpatrick and Morgan (1980, pp. 372–373) concluded, "Female homosexuality is to be understood as a unique female phenomenon, rather than a state which is either the same as or the reverse of male homosexuality." Thus, femaleness has priority over sexual orientation for lesbians.

Others agree. In the same volume, Saghir and Robins (1980, p. 290) wrote, "The similarities between male and female homosexuals are limited to their dominant sexual preferences for members of the same sex. Otherwise, the female homosexuals are more like female heterosexuals while male homosexuals are more like male heterosexuals." The significance of gender differences across sexual orientations in the Saghir and Robins (1980) study was particularly notable in matters of sexual behavior, such as in partner number, frequency of occurrence, and age of onset. These gender distinctions were especially prevalent during the years of interest in this study, the adolescent and young adult years. Compared with female heterosexuals, however, lesbians behaved more frequently in a tomboyish manner, were less interested in conventional feminine characteristics such as sexual and physical attractiveness, and displayed a greater degree of assertiveness and aggressiveness (Saghir & Robins, 1980).

There is perhaps an unrecognized—and certainly unacknowledged—political agenda in the view that women are more like women and men more like men no matter what the sexual orientation: a deemphasis of the importance that sexual orientation has for shaping the lives of lesbians and gay males. This reaction may be a pendulum response to those who advocate the overriding impact—usually negative—homosexuality has on the lives of its men and women. Historically, D'Emilio (1983) noted that psychiatrists, doctors, and scientists spoke in reassuring tones when invited to early meetings of the homosexual community, such as the Mattachine Society. Their message reinforced the idea that homosexuals were just like everyone else except in whom they chose to love. Aside from societal discrimination, sexual orientation was essentially of minimal consequence for their adjustment to society. Opposed to these "accommodationists" were the "gay liberators" who proclaimed pride in their homosexuality. Sexual orientation mattered, they argued. Perhaps the analogy is overdrawn, but I believe that those who argue for the importance of sex and who minimize sexual orientation in shaping the individual reflect this historic legacy. The current data support but cannot prove the position that sexual orientation is a significant contributor to the attitudes, interests, activities, relationships, and personality of an individual.

The primary reason that the present results cannot resolve this issue is because a heterosexual sample was not included (for the reason stated earlier that straight versus gay comparisons were not my research priority). The issue is addressed below in terms of the importance of sexual orientation and gender in accounting for the gender variations found in the present study. An alternative view, which I deem of greater significance, is that neither sex nor sexual orientation is necessarily most crucial. Rather, the relative influence of each depends on the characteristic of interest. The realization of this differentiation would appear to be a productive investigative procedure.

The reasons given for the preponderance of gender over sexual orientation are rather uniform: gender socialization during the childhood and adolescent years (Gagnon & Simon, 1973; Kirkpatrick & Morgan, 1980; Schafer, 1977; Tripp, 1975). The gender difference can be most clearly noted when comparing the two areas where the sexes diverge most profoundly in empirical investigations, namely, sexual behaviors and love affairs.

Tripp (1975) believed that homosexual males are far more sexually promiscuous than are homosexual females, who do not know the meaning of anonymous sex. Rather, lesbians are more inclined to develop intimate, meshing accords with other lesbians. The greater lasting power of lesbian love affairs is due, Tripp believed, to the " 'nest building' proclivities which permit them to extract more nonsexual rewards from a close relationship than men can" (p. 164). This difference between lesbians and gay males is shared with their heterosexual sisters and brothers. Tripp suggested that this sex difference may be due to both biological (lower libido of females) and environmental (socialization of the sexes) factors. Schafer (1977) sided with differential socialization: "Males learn from the beginning of puberty, or even earlier, to conceive of sexuality as something in and of itself and to meet these needs more independently of any affective needs they may also have" (p. 360). On the other hand, as a result of their feminine socialization, women are more likely to desire integrating their emotional and sexual lives.

Lesbians tend to have fewer sexual partners but more love affairs than gay men because they have internalized the female norm of uniting equally love and sexuality. Schafer concluded, "Thus our data would tend to indicate that being a woman tends to influence the sexual behavior of lesbians more than being a homosexual" (p. 363). This study did not, however, have a heterosexual comparison group.

In fact, however, the omission of a heterosexual comparison group is a common one. The research study investigating variations among lesbians and gay males that also includes heterosexual women and men is extremely rare. In two separate articles of perhaps questionable comparability with populations of males and females of various sexual orientations, Seigelman (1972a, 1972b) found surprisingly few differences between his homosexual and heterosexual samples in various adjustment and personality characteristics. Comparing across the two studies, there were also relatively few differences between straight and lesbian women. The largest number of differences occurred between straight and gay men. This was primarily the result of the high femininity scores of the homosexual males, who were divergent not only from the heterosexual males but also from a subsample of low-femininity homosexual males as well. Thus, the important distinction needed to better understand human behavior regardless of sex or sexual orientation is not variations between male and female or straight and gay but variations within a population itself (e.g., femininity scores for gay males).

This is exactly the point made most forcefully in terms of research by Bell and Weinberg (1978) in their book *Homosexualities: A Study of Diversity Among Men and Women:*

> *Returning to the* raison d'etre *of our study, it should be clear by now that we do not do justice to people's sexual orientation when we refer to it by a singular noun. There are "homosexualities" and there are "heterosexualities," each involving a variety of different interrelated dimensions. (p. 219. Reprinted by permission of Simon & Schuster, Inc.)*

Although they included a sample of male and female heterosexuals in their study, the results of these data are seldom discussed (they are available in the appendices). Rather, the authors were primarily concerned with typologies and variations within the sample of gay men and lesbians, with some attention given to gender differences within the homosexual population. A later book (Bell et al., 1981a), however, lost this focus. The possibility of diversity or of different routes to homosexuality implied in their first book was largely abandoned (although they do not reject the possibility of multiple pathways) in favor of a "best fit" model. The authors deemphasized the lesbian versus gay comparison and placed primary importance on straight versus gay variations by developing causal models for sexual orientation. It is disturbing, however, to note that although different male and female routes were given for adult homosexuality, apparently heterosexuality did not need explanation. Pathways to that outcome were not given, despite the generic title of the book, *Sexual Preference.*

Gay versus straight comparisons are not particularly helpful in understanding the complexities of homosexuality. For example, I am not sure why the gay youths in the present population had more homosexual sexual experiences than the lesbians. More interesting is that the difference was considerably less than that reported by others; only 10% of the males and 1% of the females had had 50 or more sexual partners. Perhaps the difference is due to the youthful age of the population (not enough time has elapsed to magnify the gender difference) or to the changing nature of homosexuality across generations (perhaps the sex in homosexuality has decreased in importance as homosexuality has become less clandestine).

Similar to other studies, lesbians had more love affairs than gay youths and the affairs lasted a longer period of time. Relatively few (14%) of the lesbians had never been in a love relationship (33% of the males never had). Because these gender differences have been well documented in heterosexual samples, one can explain the difference, with a fair amount of confidence, as derivative of gender rather than sexual orientation. But one cannot thus automatically assume, as do most researchers, on the basis of not empirical evidence but theory, that the differences in sexual behavior and love affairs are due to gender socialization forces without also examining biological, evolutionary influences.

The resolution to the fundamental issue of the relative importance of gender versus sexual orientation in accounting for behavioral and personality variations and the cause of the variations (most simplistically, biology and environment) requires additional data. Research currently available is insufficient to reach viable conclusions, although many investigators apparently believe the answer is obvious: Gender socialization explains the importance of gender over sexual orientation. Most probably, the relative centrality of gender and sexual orientation and of biology and socialization will vary as a direct function of the particular behavior or personality characteristic under consideration. For example, if lesbian relationships are more intimate than gay relationships, it is probably the result of gender rather than sexual orientation. Both socialization theorists (e.g., Gagnon & Simon, 1973) and evolutionary biologists (e.g., Freedman, 1979) offer convincing arguments to account for this gender difference.

On the other hand, the high prevalence of cross-sex friends among lesbian and gay youths appears to be more highly related to the sexual orientation than to the sex of the individual. Again, either socialization (feeling more comfortable with cross-sex members because sexual pressures are reduced) or biological (seeking friendships with other-sex individuals because of behavioral and dispositional similarities) explanations are viable. This study does not provide answers to this debate, but it does give an additional source of information, a population of lesbians and gay males seldom tapped by researchers, to future socialization- and biology-oriented investigators and theorists.

In highlighting gender differences among the youths in the current sample, it is apparent that the lesbians were more politically liberal, sports oriented, comfortable with their homosexuality, inclined to have been and currently be in a love affair, and likely to stay in a love affair. Compared with gay youths they had more sex and friendships with females, were more heterosexually experienced, more often reported that having close female friends was important for their sense of self-worth, and more frequently described themselves as athletic and understanding. Gay youths were more religious, claimed to be more exclusively homosexual, read more gay periodicals, felt gay at an earlier age, reported more frequently that their sexual orientation was beyond their control, had more sex and friendships with males, described themselves as more muscular, and reported more frequently that having close male friends, physical looks, material possessions, and religion were important for their sense of self-worth. There were no gender differences on many other variables, such as socializing with other lesbians and gays, bar attendance, number of heterosexual and bisexual friends, acceptance from family members, and most of the personality and self-worth characterizations.

These gender differences were somewhat dependent on the age of the respondents, especially the self-descriptions and sense of self-worth variables. For example, the youngest male adolescents felt more accomplished than did the youngest females; the oldest females were more likely than the oldest males to report that the parents were important for their sense of self-worth.

The data in this chapter are suggestive, but they need further investigation with a larger sample of lesbians and gay males and a longitudinal design in order to derive developmental path distinctions for females and males. Although the sexes did not vary on the sociodemographic variables, one cannot assume that they were equally representative of their sexual orientation/sex group or that they did not differ in ways not measured (e.g., developmental history and availability to social scientists). Clearly, additional studies are necessary with other samples of lesbian and gay youths.

In terms of predicting self-esteem level, summarized in Chapter 6, the sexes did not diverge drastically. Sociodemographic factors, attitudes and interests, and gay-related activities and attitudes were not significant predictors of self-esteem level for either sex. Feeling support from an accepting family and having a large number of bisexual friends were significant predictors of the lesbian youths' self-esteem. For males, having a large number of love affairs, currently being in love affair, and having had a large percentage of homosexual affairs, especially the initial one, were highly related to self-esteem level. High self-esteem youths were not shy and, if male, felt accomplished and self-sufficient. Gay males who devalued their possessions, physical looks, and frequency of sexual activities and who were oriented toward career and academic success had the highest levels of self-esteem.

In the final chapter a further portrait of the youths is presented that focuses not so much on group mean level differences and similarities as on the diversity within the lesbian and gay youth population. This discussion leads to the final concern of this book: the problems and promises of lesbian and gay youth.

10

Moving the Invisible to Visibility

OVERVIEW

The manner in which homosexuality is viewed by lesbian and gay youth, their parents and friends, and the society in which they live has both psychological and sociopolitical implications. Discussion of these issues should be a top priority, and my focus is on the visibility of lesbian and gay youth and on keeping them in mind as we develop programs and support services for the lesbian and gay communities.

Unfortunately, the visibility that lesbian and gay youth have thus far received has been primarily in the realm of the negative. That is, the focus has been on the problems and seldom the promise of gay and lesbian youth. This attention is gratifying in terms of addressing psychological well-being and physical health (e.g., acquired immune deficiency syndrome [AIDS]) issues, but short sighted in terms of the potential political ramifications. This dilemma pervades the discussion in this chapter, which reviews two political perspectives of the nature of homosexuality and homosexual persons, the diversity rather than the uniformity of lesbian and gay persons, current cultural biases against homosexuality, and the problems of lesbian and gay youth growing toward maturity in this cultural context. I close the chapter with a minority perspective, one that is most true to the data reported in this book and to the reality of the vast majority of lesbian and gay youth: the promise of gay and lesbian youth.

VIEWS OF HOMOSEXUALITY

A Central Dichotomy

The classic dichotomy of homosexuality and homosexual persons is perhaps most vividly articulated in Gloria Naylor's (1982) *The Women of Brewster Place*. Lorraine wanted most in life to be viewed as acceptable in the black community on Brewster Place:

> *No, it wasn't her job she feared losing this time, but their approval. She wanted to stand out there and chat and trade makeup secrets and cake recipes. (p. 136)*

Theresa, her lover, had a different perspective: "I personally don't give a shit what they're thinking. And their good evenings don't put any bread on my table" (p. 134). Their conflict is one that is historically characteristic of gay women and men encountering straight society.

> *"And we're just a couple of dykes." She spit the words into the air.*
> *Lorraine started as if she'd been slapped. "That's a filthy thing to say, Tee. You can call yourself that if you want to, but I'm not like that. Do you hear me? I'm not!" She slammed the*

drawer shut. . . . "When I'm with Ben, I don't feel any different from anybody else in the world."

"Then he's doing you an injustice," Theresa snapped, "because we are different. And the sooner you learn that, the better off you'll be. . . . You're a lesbian—do you understand that word?—a butch, a dyke, a lesbo, all those things that kid was shouting. Yes, I heard him! And you can run in all the basements in the world, and it won't change that, so why don't you accept it?"

"I have accepted it!" Lorraine shouted. "I've accepted it all my life, and it's nothing I'm ashamed of. I lost a father because I refused to be ashamed of it—but it doesn't make me any different from anyone else in the world."

"It makes you damned different!"

"No!" She jerked open the bottom drawer of her dresser and took out a handful of her underwear. "Do you see this? There are two things that have been a constant in my life since I was sixteen years old—beige bras and oatmeal. The day before I first fell in love with a woman, I got up, had oatmeal for breakfast, put on a beige bra, and went to school. The day after I fell in love with that woman, I got up, had oatmeal for breakfast, and put on a beige bra. I was no different the day before or after that happened, Tee."

"And what did you do when you went to school that next day, Lorraine? Did you stand around the gym locker and swap stories with the other girls about this new love in your life, uh?" (G. Naylor, *The Women of Brewster Place*, pp. 164–165. Copyright © 1980, 1982, by Gloria Naylor. Reprinted by permission of Viking Penguin.)

These two perspectives carry political weight because of the consequences that each has had historically and will have in future discussions. Advocating the view that gay men and women are just like everyone else, except for whom they choose to love, will play, I believe, nicely to those who fear us, are uncomfortable with us, and want us to disappear. It is a conservative, fitting-in position that D'Emilio referred to as accommodation. Historically, there have been gay men and lesbians and organizations (e.g., after the advent of Harry Hay's Mattachine Society) who pursued the acceptance of homosexuality by mainstream society, especially the professional segments such as medicine and law, at any cost. If we acted or looked a little strange it was not because of any deficit inherent in our biological makeup but because of persecution and discrimination encountered both directly and indirectly through societal attitudes and stereotypes. If you treat us respectably then we will be normal, good citizens with civic responsibilities and appropriate behaviors.

At times the real enemy for the accommodationists appears to be the radicals or the gay liberators rather than the persecutors of gay persons in straight society. According to this view, the gay liberators provide the wrong image at the wrong time, exemplifying what our friends in straight society fear most: confusing sex roles, presenting dykes and queens as members of the community, advocating the sexual rights of minors, and threatening the social and political system.

The gay radical perspective maintains that by definition gay women and men are "atypical." This may be due to the biology that creates our sexual orientation and perhaps other facets of personality (e.g., gender-atypical postures and gestures, sensitivity, artistic talent) or to the environment, such as the oppression that a gay person inevitably experiences or fears encountering. Radicals emphasizing the biologic origins of the atypicality are likely to advocate that society ought to broaden its acceptance levels such that the "biologically normal" includes the full spectrum from exclusively homosexual to exclusively heterosexual. Masculinity and femininity, from this perspective, should be unhinged from biological sex and be perceived as characteristics of persons, to varying degrees. The environmentally biased radicals see little immediate hope that society will change its oppressive nature. Many do not request acceptance of lesbian and gay life-styles, but do demand civil rights and an end to verbal and physical violence.

Diversity

On one topic both accommodationists and radicals would agree: There is diversity among gay people. Until recently an unspoken assumption in traditional research on homosexuality has been that all gay people are essentially very much alike. Fortunately, several researchers have addressed the heterogeneity within the lesbian and gay population. For example, Bell and Weinberg's (1978) book, *Homosexualities*, exploded the myth of homosexual conformity with an emphasis on within-group variations. This resulted in a presentation of various portraits of gay and lesbian adults that have been discussed throughout this book. However, few social scientists, health care providers, or members of the mass media have listened. As a result, cognizance of the diversity within the lesbian and gay population has been preempted by examining characteristics thought to distinguish homosexual from heterosexual people. This focus has not been pursued in this book, for reasons noted in Chapter 1.

One source of diversity is age. Gay and lesbian youth may be developmentally quite different from adults, both gay and straight, but, according to an accommodation perspective, they may be in many important ways similar to other adolescents. For example, lesbian and gay youths internalize and incorporate, to some degree, into their self-image the perceptions of others, such as family members. Thus, if parents reject their daughter or son because of her or his sexual orientation, then the adolescent may also reject herself or himself and develop low self-esteem (see Chapter 8). On the other hand, this rejection may be one more example, from a radical perspective, of the necessary uniqueness of being young and gay and the oppression that gay and lesbian youth inevitably face.

Focusing on diversity had intriguing repercussions in Boxer's (1988) research. He noted two pathways of initiation into sexual identity formation among Chicago gay youths. The mean age of first same-sex activity for 75% of the males was 15.0 years; all had begun homosexual activity after the age of 11 years. The other cluster of males (25%) reported that their first same-sex activity, usually with a same-aged peer, occurred prior to age 9 years ($M = 6.5$ years). The implications of these two tracks have yet to be sorted but they may have significance in terms of psychological well-being and coming out. Research that treats all gay and lesbian youth as if they were engaged in identical developmental pathways may be obscuring important developmental processes and outcomes.

Even if it proves to be the case that sexual orientation per se produces important differences in developmental outcomes, far more studies that focus on unique patterns among those with a homosexual sexual orientation are needed. By this methodology gay people are treated not as removed from the "developmentally normal" but as a unique (whether for biological and/or socialization reasons) population that needs to be understood on its own terms and with its own diversities. With this effort social scientists increase the likelihood of learning about development in all of its manifestations.

As researchers we seem bent, however, on emphasizing gay versus straight comparisons, a mentality that is also reflected in the larger culture. For example, Russo (1987) noted that the dominant culture frequently makes films about homosexuality to illustrate how homosexuals differ from heterosexuals. He demanded, "No more films about homosexuality" (p. 326). Taken for granted in many films is that being gay is by definition odd or erotic. What he felt was needed were:

> Films that explore people who happen to be gay in America and how their lives intersect with the dominant culture. . . . Gay sensibility [is] a blindness to sexual divisions, an inability to perceive that people are different simply because of sexuality, a natural conviction that difference exists but doesn't matter. (The Celluloid Closet, p. 326. Reprinted by permission of Harper & Row.)

Prick Up Your Ears, Maurice, and Torch Song Trilogy would probably be more acceptable movies for Russo because they primarily explore issues of identity, interpersonal attraction, and societal oppression with characters who happen to be gay. Whether the perspective is accommodation or radicalism, viewing homosexuality as developmentally unique or similar to heterosexuality may be less important than attempting to understand the experience of being young and gay in the United States, bringing that experience to public visibility, and helping gay and lesbian youth lead creative and happy lives.

Diversity in the Current Sample

The youths in this study were neither representative of the total gay and lesbian youth population nor randomly derived, as noted in Chapter 4. Although a diverse group of youths was included, there were relatively few young adolescents, ethnic minorities, and unschooled youths. Despite the efforts of the female research assistants, my attempt to increase the number of lesbians in the study proved frustrating. This shortage may reflect (a) the lower number of gay women than men in the population, as noted historically by Kinsey, Pomeroy, Martin, and Gebhard (1953) and more recently by Bell, Weinberg, and Hammersmith (1981a), or, as the literature also indicates (e.g., de Monteflores & Schultz, 1978), (b) the tendency for lesbians to come out at a later age (after late adolescence) than gay males.

On the other hand, the overall diversity of the current sample is supported by the inclusion of individuals seldom appearing in previous studies of gay males and lesbians of any age: adolescents under the age of 18 years; those with 12 or fewer years of education; gay persons from rural areas, small towns, and working class homes; those who express significant heterosexual interest; and youths not yet out to anyone or out to few others. Future research needs to expand our knowledge of young gays and lesbians from a variety of backgrounds, behaviors, and attitudes. With a larger and more diverse population of youths, future studies will begin to untangle the significance of these characteristics, not only for issues addressed in this book, but for many others as well.

The evolution of identity among lesbian and gay youth is an issue of particular interest to me. A focus on identity development requires research that extends empirical investigations beyond the evaluative dimension of the self (i.e., self-esteem) to other components of the self-concept among gay males and lesbians. Needed are in-depth, longitudinal studies that trace qualitatively the evolving sense of self as a gay or lesbian person from the first moments of cognition in infancy and childhood to its full recognition and acceptance during maturity. The perceptual and cognitive aspects of a gay or lesbian identity are little understood.

GAY AND LESBIAN YOUTH AS PROBLEMATIC

The Evolution of Difficulties

The classical "storm and stress" perspective of adolescence is viewed by some as particularly pertinent for gay and lesbian adolescents, for theoretical reasons noted in Chapter 2. For example, sociological theories maintain that the social environment (family, peers, and cultural traditions) exerts inordinate influence during childhood and adolescence as the pre-gay or pre-lesbian youth strives to discover a sexual identity within a social context. Frequently, these influences attempt to deny the very definition of that which feels most natural. Rigg, a physician, noted the possible negative repercussions of this experience (1982, p. 827):

As time passes and the realization comes that the homosexual drive is not being dispelled, but is becoming stronger, an identity crisis may occur which may be handled in a variety of ways, and therefore may be associated with varied new symptoms. The most obvious one is depression, which may be manifested by withdrawal, lack of interest in schoolwork, lack of interest in activities which involve associating with peers, irritability and moodiness. Loss of peer relationships naturally produces a sense of isolation, which heightens the fear of abandonment already present and increases depression.

A retrospective study (Bell et al., 1981a) supported this view: More gay than non-gay males and females recalled feeling anxious, insecure, frustrated, and miserable during their adolescence. As adults they recalled that they were often socially submissive, passive, and weak when interacting with others. In the Netherlands, G. Sanders (1980) noted that gay youth, compared with straight youth, are more likely to experience difficulties in finding positive models and confidants. Accurate information concerning their sexual identity and how they should integrate with peers is missing, thus thrusting them into periods of conflict.

The child learns quite early that homosexuality must be wrong, sick, and certainly undesirable.

A major crisis is created for the individual, the family, and ultimately for society when a child appears about to break with these expectations. Minimally, the child feels different, alienated, and alone. As they grow up, many such children develop low self-esteem. If acknowledged, same-sex feelings would mean rejection and ridicule; consequently, individuals protect themselves from awareness through defenses, such as denial, repression, reaction formation, sublimation, and rationalization. . . . The consequences of this concealment can be enormously destructive. (Coleman, 1982, p. 33)

By adolescence, according to this view, the individual has learned that he or she is among the most despised and is thus faced with a number of decisions at a time when one is least able to make the right choices (Martin, 1982). Malyon (1981, p. 324) noted, that intrapsychic conflict with one's homoerotic impulses in combination with social disapproval may have dire consequences:

Homophobic content becomes internalized and often causes protracted dysphoria and feelings of self-contempt. The juxtaposition of homosexual desire and acculturated self-criticism is inimical to healthy psychological development.

In family relations they become half-members: "afraid and alienated, unable ever to be totally open and spontaneous, to trust or be trusted, to develop a fully socialized sense of self-affirmation . . . stress characterized by secrecy, ignorance, helplessness, and distance" (MacDonald, 1983, p. 1). The "secret" must be hidden—from peers, family, and self—as the adolescent learns and feels the wisdom of invisibility and dishonesty.

These conflicts may be expressed in childhood and adolescence through various behavioral problems such as acting out in school, rebellion against authority, substance abuse, prostitution, and suicide and feelings of depression, isolation, confusion, and alienation (Robertson, 1981; Rutter, 1980). More common, however, are subtle, "small hurts" that occur whenever lesbians and gay men believe they cannot fully express their true thoughts and feelings. Fisher (1972, p. 249) noted that "The effect may be scarcely noticeable: joy may be a little less keen, happiness slightly subdued; he may simply feel a little run down, a little less tall. Over the years, these tiny denials have a cumulative effect."

If a youth takes the courageous step of coming out as lesbian or gay, a number of dire consequences may result. Ostracism, violence, and expulsion by peers and family may face her or him. Many of the youths in Remafedi's (1987a) research reported that they were victims of physical assaults (30%), had been discriminated against in education and employment (37%), received regular verbal abuse from peers (55%), and saw disadvantages to being gay (100%). The most frequent psychosocial and medical problems were, in order, poor school performance (80% of those in school), mental health problems (72%), substance abuse (58%), running away (48%), and conflict with the law (48%) (Remafedi, 1987b).

One concern that appears to reach its developmental peak during adolescence is status among peers. Maintaining intimacy, trust, self-disclosure, and loyalty in friendships is a major developmental task of adolescence (Savin-Williams & Berndt, 1990), yet youths are equally concerned that these same-sex relationships not be viewed as sexually intimate (Eder & Sanford, 1986). They fear the rumors and the consequences. Anti-gay bashings, ridicule, and violence are frequently perpetuated by young men in their teens and early 20s, as several grisly accounts in New York City illustrate (Harding, 1988). Both gay and lesbian youths have received a renewed wave of violence with the AIDS crisis. Hunter, at the Hetrick-Martin Institute, reported that lesbian and gay youths have been called an "AIDS factory" by their peers (Freiberg, 1987). According to *The Advocate* (Peterson, 1988), one Seattle youth testified before a city commission, "I dropped out of school when I was 16 because of the harassment I faced there. I was beat up after school. My lockers were trashed. I was also harassed by teachers at the school I attended." The *Washington Post* reported Stuart Reges's story of attempted suicide midway through his senior year in high school: "I was a young gay person desperately trying to be a young non-gay person, and I couldn't accept my failure" (Murdoch, 1988, p. A1). It was the threat of being isolated and alienated from peers that contributed to his decision to end his life.

Psychological and social services are seldom available to lesbian and gay youth as they attempt to establish a sense of inner and outer identity. Few parents are willing to consent to psychotherapeutic services unless the ultimate treatment goal is conversion to heterosexuality (Malyon, 1981). Most established lesbian and gay male cultural activities and institutions are for adults only (see Chapter 1). Malyon (1981, p. 328) reviewed these issues and pointed out: "Self-acknowledged homosexual adolescents, then, are often an alienated and neglected population. The personal, social, and institutional support systems that assist the adolescent heterosexual minor are not available to the homosexual minor. As might be expected, this situation often produces rather morbid psychological consequences."

Many youths must therefore attempt to be adolescents in a "hostile and psychologically impoverished heterosexual" social world (Malyon, 1981, p. 325). Some lesbian and gay youth, though primarily only in large urban areas, find psychological support services that help them cope with discrimination and homophobic attitudes and develop a positive, fulfilling life-style (e.g., the Sexual Minority Youth Assistance League in Washington, DC). A growing number of mental health professionals refuse to "treat" men and women who wish to change their sexual orientation. All too frequently, however, these services and professionals are available only to adults and not to adolescents.

The school system has certainly contributed to difficulties encountered by lesbian and gay youth. An unfortunate prototypical example is the state of sex education in the public schools and the community. Freiberg reviewed these issues in a 1987 article in *The Advocate*, "Sex Education and the Gay Issue: What Are They Teaching About Us in the Schools?" Homosexuality and emotional relations among same-sex individuals are almost universally ignored in sex education curricula. Teachers fear the negative reactions of parents and the school board and the community furor that inclusion of homosexuality in school classes would create. Unfortunately, AIDS education frequently carries the message "Look how unhealthy homosexuality is." Because most instigators of anti-gay tormenting have recently been in the public school system, an educational opportunity has generally been lost (Freiberg, 1987).

At Mead High School in Spokane, Washington, both a teacher, Ted Ketcham, and a 17-year-old male gay student discovered the consequences of addressing gay issues at school (Peterson, 1989a). The verbally and physically harassed student was asked by Ketcham to speak to his classmates about being gay. The session went poorly, parents began a letter-writing campaign to protest open discussion of homosexuality, and the name-calling and threats of violence against the student forced him to leave school. Ketcham was disciplined by the school district, but the latter in turn was chastized for not disciplining the harassers and for being unprepared to address issues of homosexuality.

The mental health and educational deficiencies are due in part, it seems, to the invisibility of lesbian and gay adolescents in society at large. This invisibility contributes to a sense of alienation and stress for the individual adolescent that is frequently noted by various theoretical models and occasionally by empirical evidence, and yet is denied by those concerned with the education and health of adolescents. Lesbian and gay youth are uniquely at risk and thus in need of access to intervention and support programs.

Winds of Change?

Despite the fact that striking changes have occurred in the United States during the past decade in terms of the visibility of lesbians and gay men, it is instructive to note that many past, antihomosexual theories and treatment approaches remain as part of the belief system of a considerable number of professionals. A review by

Schwanberg (1985) noted that this is most pronounced in psychiatry and less so in psychology, medicine, nursing, and the social sciences. Almost exclusively, however, these conceptualizations have focused on adult sexual behavior, with only occasional reference to adolescents. Nonetheless, these general theories necessarily influence the education and training of health care personnel and consequently the forms of health care and intervention strategies used in contacts with gay and non-gay adolescents.

Cultural shifts are becoming evident, however. For example, in 1969 the medical journal *Pediatrics* recognized the importance of adolescent homosexuality for scientific and humanistic reasons, but it was considered to be a "developmental deviance" (Solnit, 1969). Fourteen years later in 1983 the position of the American Academy of Pediatrics, Committee on Adolescence (1983), was quite different: Homosexuality as a sexual orientation is established before adolescence, homosexual behavior is common even for those who become conventionally heterosexual, homosexual behavior may occur given particular environmental contexts (e.g., incarceration, single sex boarding schools, military barracks), and problems with homosexuality are usually the consequence of social conditions rather than of mental illness. The necessity for a positive attitude on the part of the pediatrician was emphasized:

> *The pediatrician must be entirely non-judgmental in posing sexual questions if he or she is to be at all effective in encouraging the teenager to share his or her concerns, experiences, and beliefs. Only with adequate information of this kind can there be proper medical assessment of the potential consequences of homosexual practice or fears. If the history includes open-ended questions about homosexual beliefs, practices, and experiences, then the pediatrician may elicit items that require either further investigation and evaluation, or possibly referral. (pp. 249–250)*

If the pediatrician is unable to be nonjudgmental, then patients should be referred to someone who can be. The physician's responsibility is to

> *. . . provide health care for homosexual adolescents and guidance for those young people struggling with problems of sexual expression. The pediatrician can play a role in the evaluation and care of those adolescents who are concerned about their expression of sexual preference by offering reassurance to those in discomfort because of early adolescent homosexual experience; willingness to help or refer for help those in difficulty with family, peers, or institutions; and by being familiar with community resources for teenaged homosexuals and their parents if referral for social and emotional stress is required. (p. 250. Reproduced by permission of Pediatrics.)*

The Toronto Board of Education recently voted to combat homophobic bias and violence through a sex education program. Educators at Santa Clara County, California, proposed a school-based counseling program for lesbian and gay youth, with a designated gay-sensitive adult in each secondary school. A Seattle commission recommended that accurate, objective, and relevant information concerning sexual orientation be taught in the school system's family life courses and that a gay-sensitive staff member be made available in each middle and senior high school (similar to the San Francisco school system). New York City's Harvey Milk School for lesbian and gay youth is firmly established 5 years after its beginning with some 40 students enrolled per year. For these lesbian and gay youth, school is now a safe place where both education and personal healing can occur with lesbian and gay teachers and social workers and a curriculum that highlights the positive contributions of lesbians and gay men to world history and culture. A student praised the staff: "I didn't expect everyone to be so nice and so caring. They really care about what you're doing and what you want to become in the future" (Freiberg, 1989).

Our culture needs to realize that the adjustment problems experienced by many lesbian and gay youth are due not so much to developmental defects that are inherent within the individual but to societal defects that cause individual pathology. McDonald (1982) elaborated the point by noting, in reference to coming out, that this critical identity issue usually occurs in an antihomosexual environment without institutional or social support:

> *What coming out ultimately symbolizes is the individuals' response to social stigmatization in a struggle to redefine him/herself against a background of antihomosexual prejudice and discrimination. Only with reconstruction of social conditions and attitudes will individuals experience, with pride and dignity, an integration of their feelings, behavior, and identity into a unified and positive self-concept. (p. 58)*

Social attitudes toward lesbians and gay men, however, remain negative, primarily because they serve the status quo of traditional sex roles, behaviors, and morality (Herek, 1984; Morin & Garfinkle, 1978). A Gallup Poll (1982) indicated that the American public views homosexuals, by a 5 to 1 margin, as less likely than heterosexuals to lead happy, well-adjusted lives and, by a 2 to 1 margin, as more likely to have drug and alcohol problems.

Surveying 278 high school students, Price (1982) found a high degree of antihomosexual attitudes when the issue was personal, potentially affecting the youths directly. For example, the youths strongly endorsed the following views: "As a parent I would be upset if my child was homosexual," "The thought of homosexuality makes me sick," "I would not have a close friend who was homosexual," and "I do not want to live close to a homosexual." On the other hand, they were relatively neutral in regard to whether homosexuals should be allowed to hold important jobs, are criminals and should be locked up, and should be recognized as similar to everyone else. Male adolescents held more negative attitudes than did female youths. These findings were essentially a replication of earlier studies of adolescent attitudes toward homosexuality (Sobel, 1976; Sorensen, 1973).

There is some evidence, however, that these negative attitudes are beginning to shift among adolescents, at least among economically, educationally, and socially privileged adolescents (Savin-Williams, 1989c). In a survey of 356 youths who had just completed their junior year in high school (age range = 16 to 18 years), the privileged adolescents were clearly more liberal than the general population in regard to the civil rights of lesbians and gay men, including their rights to engage in homosexual sex. For example, more than 80% believed that a gay person should be allowed to teach in college or speak in the community, and only 32% said that homosexual sex was always wrong. Comparable percentages among adults were 58%, 67%, and 73%, respectively. This tolerance was restricted, however, to civil rights. It was seldom extended to personal encounters such as feeling comfortable with a homosexual person moving into one's neighborhood, inviting a homosexual to dinner, and having a homosexual relative.

Rofes (1984) was not particularly optimistic with the current plight of gay and lesbian adolescents in today's society:

While some of us imagine a drastically changing world for gay teens, this appears to be more an activist's fantasy than reality. Gay teens still feel isolated in their homes, neighborhoods, and schools. It's a rare gay teenager who finds support in his or her high school—either from another gay student or an openly gay teacher.

The options for the typical gay teenager in high school really haven't expanded much after 15 years of the contemporary gay and lesbian movement. (p. 15)

On the other hand, as the social–historical and cohort time frames change, so too may the experiences of the adolescent coming to terms with same-sex feelings, attractions, and behaviors. Learning to cope with these feelings frequently involves keeping homosexuality a secret, perhaps from oneself and certainly from others. After all, who admits or declares publicly their sexual orientation when that very existence is deemed immoral or mentally ill? Gay and lesbian youth are engulfed in a culture in which antihomosexual attitudes proliferate. Pre-gay and pre-lesbian youth may be wise to worry about exposure and anticipate discrimination. Consequently, they may understandably choose to hide their sexual orientation, which may in turn result in a variety of psychological problems. One can hope that a liberating trend that encourages a diversity of sexual expressions at all ages is emerging. Indeed, it would appear that today's adolescents are arriving at a homosexual identification and engaging in homosexual behavior at earlier ages (McDonald, 1982; Rigg, 1982; Robinson, 1984; Smith, 1983). Now what is needed are adults and peers who will listen, accept, and support these youths as they discover their natural and enduring self.

THE PROMISE OF LESBIAN AND GAY YOUTH

Although the portrait presented in the preceding section may represent some gay and lesbian youths, many others accept their homosexual feelings and attractions and lead successful, productive, nonneurotic lives as self-acknowledged gay men and lesbians. But social scientists, including lesbian and gay researchers, have focused almost exclusively on the "problems" at the expense of the "promises" of lesbian and gay youth. It is perhaps surprising that the results of the current study presented lesbian and gay adolescents as essentially psychologically and socially healthy individuals. This would also appear to be the prognosis among Boxer's (1988) youths who reported relatively few negative feelings (30% of the girls and 20% of the boys) surrounding first same-sex attractions and fantasies. First homosexual activity elicited even lower levels of negative feelings among the girls (15%) and only slightly higher levels for the boys (25%). Remafedi (1987a) as well reported that his 29 youths were self-accepting and satisfied with their lives. Given the choice, 15 said they would make no change in their sexuality.

The negative portrait is the result of two groups who have been traditionally concerned with gay and lesbian youth. First, sociologists of deviance have focused on deviants and their identity problems and subcultural life-styles. Although most researchers who assume a social labeling perspective encourage tolerance ("They are at least as good as anyone else"), by their comparisons with "normals" the implicit message is clear: Gay men and lesbians are outside normalcy. The best example of this research, studies that compare the self-esteem of homosexuals with that of heterosexuals, was noted in Chapter 2. Liazos (1980) maintained that researchers need to focus far more attention on the oppressors and persecutors of homosexuality—they are indeed the deviants.

The second group are the clinicians and those in the helping professions who usually encounter lesbian and gay youths in crisis. Hippler vowed in his 1986 article in *The Advocate* that he would address both the promise and the problem of gay youth. In reality, however, the article was devoted almost entirely to the latter—primarily, I suspect, because the author's sources were clinicians, counselors, therapists, and youth workers. Although these professionals are beginning the crucial task of offering services to lesbian and gay youth in trouble with parents, the law, drugs, and themselves, they are not likely to provide a well-rounded portrait. But to be fair, social scientists have provided few other sources from which to draw another perspective.

Perhaps the most frequently quoted and referenced writings on the problems of lesbian and gay adolescents have been produced by the staff at the Hetrick-Martin Institute for the Protection of Lesbian and Gay Youth in New York City (e.g., Martin, 1982). A recent summary of this problem-focused perspective is Hetrick and Martin's (1987) article, "Developmental Issues and Their Resolution for Gay and Lesbian Adolescents." They cited the problems of social identity, stigmatization, and coping strategies that lesbian and gay adolescents confront when they hear negative verbal statements (e.g., "faggot" and "dyke"), face discriminations (legal, social, and personal), and experience violence (physical and psychological). They are socially, emotionally, and cognitively isolated, especially from the family:

> *They may feel afraid to show friendship for a friend of the same sex for fear of being misunderstood or giving away their secretly held sexual orientation; they may feel emotionally distanced and isolated from their families because they must be on guard at all times. (Hetrick & Martin, 1987, p. 31)*

Other presenting problems included suicide, sexual abuse, drug use, and depression. Over time the adolescent develops coping strategies, but the ones reviewed were primarily maladaptive: learning to hide through deception and self-monitoring, denial of membership, identification with the dominant (heterosexual) group, self-fulfilling negativism, and gender deviance (e.g., cross-dressing). Outcomes frequently included anxiety, alienation, self-hatred, and demoralization. Not until the last page of the Hetrick and Martin article is there a reference to the fact that homosexually oriented youth may have a positive ("resilience") characteristic: Homosexuality does not "invariably lead to unhappiness" (p. 40). Lesbian and gay adolescents vary in their ability to react to and handle problems, but passing through adolescence is not presented as a positive experience.

This "clinicalization" of adolescence is not unique to gay and lesbian youth; it is a battle that is fought on all fronts in mainstream developmental psychology (Savin-Williams, 1987a). This negative, problem-centered approach, however, distorts our view. For example, Martin (quoted in Hippler, 1986, p. 57) stated, "For most gay youth in this country things have not changed at all in the last 10 or 15 years." This point is highly debatable—if nothing else, the visibility and hence option of homosexuality have permeated much of American culture.

Gay and lesbian youth are, with increasing frequency, coming out during their adolescence with great portent of positive outcomes.

> *The opening of closets and the freedom which attends this event even now reveals teenagers who are fully aware of their sexual orientation as homosexuals. These young gays are refusing*

to hide who they are. In previously unsupportive environments such as parochial schools and military families, these children are now standing up for their rights; they are affirming their sexual identities as a positive force in their lives. (Uhrig, 1984, p. 117)

Occasionally this may take a quite visible form. For example, Sloan Chase Wiesen, editor of his prep school newspaper, the *Montclair Kimberley Academy News*, published a full-page editorial, "Mythcontheptions About Being Gay," during his senior year in high school. Topics covered included homophobia, coming out, AIDS, stereotypes, resources, and recommended readings. He closed with the following:

There are no men, no women, no gays, no straights; there are only people who should be free to engage in the beautiful and harmless expression of romantic love to whomever they are drawn. Be yourself, whether that means being homosexual, bisexual, or heterosexual. If you are not yet sure what you are, that's fine too. Some people become aware of their sexuality as toddlers, some as pre-teens, some as teenagers, and even some as adults. So don't panic if you are still unsure, but never be afraid or ashamed to explore who you are and to be yourself. The only road to certain unhappiness is to pretend to be who you are not. Whatever your sexuality, you will find many others who are like you. Happy Valentine's Day. (Wiesen, 1987, p. 2)

An essay on the experience of being gay is also a topic worthy of college admission forms. One of my Cornell freshmen advisees, William Perez, recounted his experience of publicly coming out not only to his peers but, more importantly, to himself:

I'll never forget the day I was in the school lunchroom by myself. . . . One of the boys got up and walked towards me. He was tall, strong and looked straight at my face with cool, gray eyes. I sensed trouble and tried to appear oblivious to his presence, thinking that if I didn't appear afraid he would leave me alone. He put his face in my line of vision and asked, "Are you a faggot?" My heart pounded and sweat broke out profusely. What was I to do? My eyes met his and for a second I choked on my words. "No, I am not a faggot. I am gay," I finally said. An uncomfortable silence settled in, and suddenly he let out his loud laughter. He continued to laugh with his friends, and they all shot insults at me to wear me down. I stayed in my seat silently but firmly. I didn't have to say anything. Pride gave me the courage to remain seated, and I was fortunate not to have suffered anything more than harsh words. Towards the end of the lunch break, I began to walk out slowly with the realization that I'll always have to stand and fight for my individuality, regardless of the consequences. (W. Perez, personal communication, 1987)

These examples are not meant to imply that youth in trouble, for example, those who come to the Gay and Lesbian Community Services Center in Los Angeles, are not real or that their problems are not real. Consider that

65% of gay runaways . . . encountered physical or sexual abuse in their homes, 80% said they are involved in prostitution, 95% said they have problems with drugs, alcohol, or both, and almost 60% said they have attempted suicide. (Peterson, 1989b, p. 8)

It is more than tragic—it is inconceivable—that these youths receive so little adult attention and that many will die by their own hand or by complications arising from AIDS. Their condition is, fortunately, only part of the story. There are other examples of youths who survive, with or without support from their parents, peers, or adult lesbians and gay men. Support groups for lesbian and gay youth have formed in high schools in several urban areas (e.g., Chicago, Los Angeles, Minneapolis, New York, and San Francisco), but the rural and poor adolescent generally remains isolated. More investing in the future of lesbian and gay youth needs our attention, dollars, and commitment.

The findings of my research present a perspective of lesbian and gay youths who have, for the most part, positive self-images and who are coping remarkably well in American society. The research does not negate the experiences of youths who seek assistance. But it does present another side of being young and gay—a positive and promising period of the life course. I believe that we need to say this loudly and clearly and to support it in the pages of our professional journals and in the media, such that we and our youth can hear it and believe it.

References

Altman, D. (1982). *The Americanization of the homosexual, the homosexualization of America.* New York: St. Martin's Press.

American Academy of Pediatrics, Committee on Adolescence. (1983). Homosexuality and adolescence. *Pediatrics, 72,* 249–250.

Bakwin, H. (1968). Deviant gender-role behavior in children: Relation to homosexuality. *Pediatrics, 41,* 620–629.

Beebe, L. P. (1981). Acceptance, sexual orientation, and psychological health: A study of gay males. *Dissertation Abstracts International, 42,* 2041B.

Bell, A. (1975). Research in homosexuality: Back to the drawing board. *Archives of Sexual Behavior, 4,* 421–431.

Bell, A. P., & Weinberg, M. S. (1978). *Homosexualities: A study of diversity among men and women.* New York: Simon & Schuster.

Bell, A. P., Weinberg, M. S., & Hammersmith, S. K. (1981a). *Sexual preference: Its development in men and women.* Bloomington, IN: Indiana University Press.

Bell, A. P., Weinberg, M. S., & Hammersmith, S. K. (1981b). *Sexual preference: Its development in men and women (statistical appendix).* Bloomington, IN: Indiana University Press.

Bender, V. L., Davis, Y., Glover, O., & Stapp, J. (1976). Patterns of self-disclosure in homosexual and heterosexual college students. *Sex Roles, 2,* 149–160.

Benitez, J. C. (1983). The effect of gay identity acquisition on the psychological adjustment of male homosexuals. *Dissertation Abstracts International, 43,* 3350B.

Berger, R. (1982). *Gay and gray.* Urbana, IL: University of Illinois Press.

Bergler, E. (1956). *Homosexuality: Disease or way of life?* New York: Collier.

Berzon, B., & Leighton, R. (Eds.). (1979). *Positively gay.* Millbrae, CA: Celestial Arts.

Bieber, I. (1965). Clinical aspects of male homosexuality. In J. Marmor (Ed.), *Sexual inversion: The multiple roots of homosexuality* (pp. 248–267). New York: Basic Books.

Bieber, I., Dain, H. J., Dince, P. R., Drellich, M. G., Grand, H. G., Gundlach, R. H., Kremer, M. W., Rifkin, A. H., Wilbur, C. B., & Bieber, T. B. (1962). *Homosexuality: A psychoanalytic study.* New York: Basic Books.

Bilotta, V. M. (1977). An existential–phenomenological study of gay male permanent lover relationships. *Dissertation Abstracts International, 38,* 345B.

Blumstein, P., & Schwartz, P. (1983). *American couples: Money, work, sex.* New York: Morrow.

Borhek, M. V. (1983). *Coming out to parents.* New York: Pilgrim.

Boswell, J. (1980). *Christianity, social tolerance and homosexuality.* Chicago: University of Chicago Press.

Boxer, A. M. (1988, March). *Betwixt and between: Developmental discontinuities of gay and lesbian youth.* Paper presented at the Society for Research on Adolescence, Alexandria, VA.

Boxer, A. M., & Cohler, B. J. (1989). The life course of gay and lesbian youth: An immodest proposal for the study of lives. *Journal of Homosexuality, 17,* 315–355.

Braaten, L. J., & Darling, C. D. (1956). Overt and covert homosexual problems among male college students. *Genetic Psychology Monographs, 71,* 269–310.

Brady, S. M. (1985). The relationship between differences in stages of homosexual identity formation and background characteristics, psychological well-being and homosexual adjustment. *Dissertation Abstracts International, 45,* 3328B.

Brooks-Gunn, J. (1987). Pubertal processes and girls' psychological adaptation. In R. M. Lerner & T. T. Foch (Eds.), *Biological–psychosocial interactions in early adolescence* (pp. 123–154). Hillsdale, NJ: Lawrence Erlbaum.

Brown, D. G. (1957). The development of sex-role inversion and homosexuality. *Journal of Pediatrics, 50,* 613–619.

Bullough, V. L. (1976). *Sexual variance in society and history.* Chicago: University of Chicago Press.

Caprio, F. S. (1954). *Female homosexuality: A psychodynamic study of lesbianism.* New York: Citadel.

Carlson, H. M., & Steuer, J. (1985). Age, sex-role categorization, and psychological health in American homosexual and heterosexual men and women. *Journal of Social Psychology, 125,* 203–211.

Cass, V. (1979). Homosexual identity formation: A theoretical model. *Journal of Homosexuality, 4,* 219–235.

Cass, V. (1984). Homosexual identity formation: Testing a theoretical model. *Journal of Sex Research, 20,* 143–167.

Cattell, R. B., & Marony, J. H. (1962). The use of the 16 PF in distinguishing homosexuals, normals, and general criminals. *Journal of Consulting Psychology, 26,* 531–540.

Chang, J., & Block, J. (1960). A study of identification in male homosexuals. *Journal of Consulting Psychology, 24,* 307–310.

Chng, C. L. (1980). Adolescent homosexual behavior and the health educator. *Journal of School Health, 61,* 517–520.

Churchill, W. (1967). *Homosexual behavior among males.* New York: Hawthorn.

Clark, D. (1977). *Loving someone gay.* New York: Signet.

Clingman, J., & Fowler, M. G. (1976). Gender roles and human sexuality. *Journal of Personality Assessment, 40,* 276–284.

Cohen-Ross, J. L. (1985). An exploratory study of the retrospective role of significant others in homosexual identity development. *Dissertation Abstracts International, 46,* 628B.

Coleman, E. (1982). Developmental states of the coming out process. *Journal of Homosexuality, 7,* 31–43.

Coleman, E. (1987). Assessment of sexual orientation. *Journal of Homosexuality, 14,* 9–24.

Coles, R., & Stokes, G. (1985). *Sex and the American teenager.* New York: Harper & Row.

Colgan, P. (1987). Treatment of identity and intimacy issues in gay males. *Journal of Homosexuality, 14,* 101–123.

Cooley, C. H. (1912). *Human nature and the social order.* New York: Scribners.

Coopersmith, S. (1967). *The antecedents of self-esteem.* San Francisco: Freeman.

Cornett, C. W., & Hudson, R. A. (1985). Psychoanalytic theory and affirmation of the gay life style: Are they necessarily antithetical? *Journal of Homosexuality, 12,* 97–108.

Cory, D. W. (1951). *The homosexual in America.* New York: Greenberg.

Cramer, D. W. (1986). Coming out to the family: An exploration of the role of selected aspects of family functioning in the disclosure decision and outcome. *Dissertation Abstracts International, 46,* 2967A.

Dailey, D. M. (1979). Adjustment of heterosexual and homosexual couples in pairing relationships: An exploratory study. *Journal of Sex Research, 15,* 143–157.

Dall'orto, G. (1987, March 17). Lively panorama for gay people in Italy: Political identity and social integration coexist. *The Advocate,* pp. 28–33.

Dank, B. M. (1971). Coming out in the gay world. *Psychiatry, 34,* 180–197.

Dank, B. M. (1973). The homosexual. In D. Spiegel & P. Keith-Spiegel (Eds.), *Outsiders USA* (pp. 269–297). San Francisco: Rinehart.

D'Augelli, A. R., & Hart, M. M. (1987). Gay women, men, and families in rural settings: Toward the development of helping communities. *American Journal of Community Psychology, 15,* 79–93.

Davis, M. (1958). *Sex and the adolescent.* New York: Perma.

Dean, R. B., & Richardson, H. (1964). Analysis of MMPI profiles of forty college-educated overt male homosexuals. *Journal of Consulting Psychology, 28,* 483–486.

de Beauvoir, S. (1963). The lesbian. In H. M. Ruitenbeek (Ed.), *The problem of homosexuality in modern society* (pp. 227–248). New York: E. P. Dutton.

D'Emilio, J. (1983). *Sexual politics, sexual communities.* Chicago: University of Chicago Press.

Demo, D. H. (1985). The measurement of self-esteem: Refining our methods. *Journal of Personality and Social Psychology, 48,* 1490–1502.

Demo, D. H., & Savin-Williams, R. C. (1983). Early adolescent self-esteem as a function of social class: Rosenberg and Pearlin revisited. *American Journal of Sociology, 88,* 763–774.

Demo, D. H., Small, S. A., & Savin-Williams, R. C. (1987). Family relations and the self-esteem of adolescents and their parents. *Journal of Marriage and the Family, 49,* 705–715.

de Monteflores, C., & Schultz, S. J. (1978). Coming out: Similarities and differences for lesbians and gay men. *Journal of Social Issues, 34,* 59–72.

Dickey, B. A. (1961). Attitude toward sex roles and feelings of adequacy in homosexual males. *Journal of Consulting Psychology, 25,* 116–122.

Doidge, W. T., & Holtzman, W. H. (1960). Implications of homosexuality among Air Force trainees. *Journal of Consulting Psychology, 24,* 9–13.

Dorian, L. (1965). *The anatomy of a homosexual.* New York: L. S. Publications.

Duke, P. M., Litt, I. F., & Gross, R. T. (1986). Adolescents' self-assessment of sexual maturation. *Pediatrics, 66,* 918–920.

DuMas, F. M. (1979). *Gay is not good.* Nashville, TN: Thomas Nelson.

Eder, D., & Sanford, S. (1986). The development and maintenance of interactional norms among early adolescents. In P. Adler (Ed.), *Sociological studies of child development* (Vol. 1, pp. 283–300). Greenwich, CT: JAI Press.

Elliot, P. E. (1982). Lesbian identity and self disclosure. *Dissertation Abstracts International, 42,* 3494B.

Erikson, E. H. (1959). Identity and the life cycle. *Psychological Issues, 1,* 1–171.

Ettorre, E. M. (1980). *Lesbians, women and society.* London: Routledge & Kegan Paul.

Evans, R. B. (1970). Sixteen personality factor questionnaire scores of homosexual men. *Journal of Consulting and Clinical Psychology, 34,* 212–215.

Evans, R. B. (1971). Adjective Checklist scores of homosexual men. *Journal of Personality Assessment, 35,* 344–349.

Fairchild, B., & Hayward, N. (1979). *Now that you know.* New York: Harcourt Brace Jovanovich.

Fay, R. E., Turner, C. F., Klassen, A. D., & Gagnon, J. H. (1989). Prevalence and patterns of same-gender sexual contact among men. *Science, 243,* 338–348.

Ferguson, K. D., & Finkler, D. C. (1978). An involvement and overtness measure for lesbians: Its development and relation to anxiety and social zeitgeist. *Archives of Sexual Behavior, 7,* 211–227.

Fisher, P. (1972). *The gay mystique: The myth and reality of male homosexuality.* New York: Stein & Day.

Fitzpatrick, G. (1983). Self-disclosure of lesbianism as related to self-actualization and self-stigmatization. *Dissertation Abstracts International, 43,* 4143B.

Fling, S., & Manosevitz, M. (1972). Sex typing in nursery school children's play interests. *Developmental Psychology, 7,* 146–152.

Fluckiger, F. A. (1966, July). Research through a glass, darkly: An evaluation of the Bieber study on homosexuality. *The Ladder, 10,* 16–26.

Ford, C. S., & Beach, F. A. (1951). *Patterns of sexual behavior.* New York: Harper & Row.

Fox, M. (1983). The spiritual journey of the homosexual . . . and just about everybody else. In R. Nugent (Ed.), *A challenge to love: Gay and lesbian Catholics in the church* (pp. 189–204). New York: Crossroad.

Freedman, D. G. (1979). *Human sociobiology: A holistic approach.* New York: Free Press.

Freedman, M. J. (1968). *Homosexuality among women and psychological adjustment.* Unpublished doctoral dissertation, Case Western Reserve University, Cleveland, OH.

Freedman, M. J. (1971). *Homosexuality and psychological functioning.* Monterey, CA: Brooks/Cole.

Freiberg, P. (1987, September 1). Sex education and the gay issue: What are they teaching about us in the schools? *The Advocate,* pp. 42–49.

Freiberg, P. (1989, April 25). A light in the blackboard jungle. *The Advocate,* pp. 50–52.

Freud, S. (1935). Letter. Published in *American Journal of Psychiatry, 107* (1951), 786.

Freud, S. (1962). *Three essays on the theory of sexuality.* New York: Basic Books.

Friend, R. A. (1980). Gayging: Adjustment and the older gay male. *Alternative Lifestyles, 3,* 231–248.

Gadpaille, W. (1980). Cross-species and cross-cultural contributions to understanding homosexual activity. *Archives of General Psychiatry, 37,* 349–356.

Gagnon, J. H., & Simon, S. (1973). *Sexual conduct: The social sources of human sexuality.* Chicago: Aldine.

Gallup Poll. (1982, November, 8). Public still stereotypes gays as insecure, unhappy. *Syracuse Post-Standard,* p. 1.

Gecas, V., & Schwalbe, M. L. (1986). Parental behavior and adolescent self-esteem. *Journal of Marriage and the Family, 48,* 37–46.

Glasser, M. (1977). Homosexuality in adolescence. *British Journal of Medical Psychology, 50,* 217–225.

Gonsiorek, J. C. (1977). Psychological adjustment and homosexuality. *JSAS Catalog of Selected Documents in Psychology, 7,* 45.

Goode, E., & Haber, L. (1977). Sexual correlates of homosexual experience: An exploratory study of college women. *Journal of Sex Research, 13,* 12–21.

Grabert, J. C. (1985). Homosexual men and their parents: A study of self-disclosure, personality traits and attitudes toward homosexuality. *Dissertation Abstracts International, 46,* 1336B.

Gray, H., & Dressel, P. (1985). Alternative interpretations of aging among gay males. *The Gerontologist, 25,* 83–87.

Green, R. (1974). *Sexual identity conflict in children and adults.* New York: Basic Books.

Green, R. (1987). *The "sissy boys syndrome" and the development of homosexuality.* New Haven, CT: Yale University Press.

Greenberg, J. S. (1973). A study of the self-esteem and alienation of male homosexuals. *Journal of Psychology, 83,* 137–143.

Greenberg, J. S. (1976). The effects of a homophile organization on the self-esteem and alienation of its members. *Journal of Homosexuality, 1,* 313–317.

Grellert, E. A. (1982). Childhood play behavior of homosexual and heterosexual men. *Psychological Reports, 51,* 607–610.

Hall, G. S. (1904). *Adolescence: Its psychology and its relations to physiology, anthropology, sociology, sex, crime, religion, and education.* New York: Appleton.

Hammersmith, S. K. (1987). A sociological approach to counseling homosexual clients and their families. *Journal of Homosexuality, 14,* 173–190.

Hammersmith, S. K., & Weinberg, M. S. (1973). Homosexual identity: Commitment, adjustment, and significant others. *Sociometry, 36,* 56–79.

Harding, R. (1988, October 10). Antigay attacks increase in New York. *The Advocate,* p. 10.

Harry, J. (1983). Defeminization and adult psychological well-being among male homosexuals. *Archives of Sexual Behavior, 12,* 1–19.

Harry, J. (1984). *Gay couples.* New York: Praeger.

Harry, J., & DeVall, W. B. (1978). *The social organization of gay males.* New York: Praeger.

Hart, M., Roback, H., Tittler, B., Weitz, L., Walston B., & McKee, E. (1978). Psychological adjustment of nonpatient homosexuals: Critical review of the research literature. *Journal of Clinical Psychiatry, 39,* 604–608.

Hatterer, L. J. (1970). *Changing homosexuality in the male.* New York: McGraw-Hill.

Hedblom, J. H. (1973). Dimensions of lesbian sexual experience. *Archives of Sexual Behavior, 2,* 329–341.

Hedblom, J. H., & Hartman, J. (1980). Research on lesbianism: Selected effects of time, geographic location, and data collection technique. *Archives of Sexual Behavior, 9,* 217–234.

Hencken, J. D. (1982). Homosexuality and psychoanalysis: Toward a mutual understanding. In W. Paul, J. D. Weinrich, J. C. Gonsiorek, & M. E. Hotvedt (Eds.), *Homosexuality: Social, psychological, and biological issues* (pp. 121–147). Beverly Hills, CA: Sage.

Hencken, J. D. (1985). Sexual-orientation self-disclosure. *Dissertation Abstracts International, 45,* 2310B.

Herdt, G. H. (1981). *Guardians of the flutes: Idioms of masculinity.* New York: McGraw-Hill.

Herek, G. M. (1984). Beyond "homophobia": A social psychological perspective on attitudes toward lesbians and gay men. *Journal of Homosexuality, 10,* 1–21.

Heron, A. (Ed.). (1983). *One teenager in ten.* Boston: Alyson.

Herron, W. G., Kinter, T., Sollinger, I., & Trubowitz, J. (1981/1982). Psychoanalytic psychotherapy for homosexual clients: New concepts. *Journal of Homosexuality, 7,* 177–192.

Hetrick, E. S., & Martin, A. D. (1987). Developmental issues and their resolution for gay and lesbian adolescents. *Journal of Homosexuality, 14,* 25–44.

Hippler, M. (1986, September 16). The problems and promise of gay youth. *The Advocate,* pp. 42–47, 55–57.

Hoffman, M. (1968). *The gay world.* New York: Basic Books.

Hooberman, R. E. (1979). Psychological androgyny, feminine gender identity and self-esteem in homosexual and heterosexual males. *Journal of Sex Research, 15,* 306–315.

Hooker, E. A. (1957). The adjustment of the male overt homosexual. *Journal of Projective Techniques, 21,* 17–31.

Hooker, E. A. (1963). The adjustment of the male overt homosexual. In H. M. Ruitenbeek (Ed.), *The problem of homosexuality in modern society* (pp. 141–161). New York: E. P. Dutton.

Hooker, E. A. (1965). Male homosexuals and their worlds. In J. Marmor (Ed.), *Sexual inversion: The multiple roots of homosexuality* (pp. 83–107). New York: Basic Books.

Hopkins, J. (1969). The lesbian personality. *British Journal of Psychiatry, 115,* 1433–1436.

Irvin, F. S. (1988, March). *Clinical perspectives on resilience among gay and lesbian youth.* Paper presented at the Society for Research on Adolescence meetings, Alexandria, VA.

James, W. (1890). *The principles of psychology.* New York: Dover.

Jay, K., & Young, A. (Eds.). (1979). *The gay report: Lesbians and gay men speak out about sexual experiences and lifestyles.* New York: Simon & Schuster.

Jourard, S. M. (1971). *The transparent self* (2nd ed.). New York: Van Nostrand.

Kaplan, E. A. (1967). Homosexuality: A search for the ego-ideal. *Archives of General Psychiatry, 16,* 355–358.

Katz, J. (1976). *Gay American history.* New York: Avon.

Kehoe, M. (1986). Lesbians over 65: A triply invisible minority. *Journal of Homosexuality, 12,* 139–152.

Kellogg, P. (1978). Breaking up. In G. Vida (Ed.), *Our right to love: A lesbian resource book* (pp. 55–56). Englewood, NJ: Prentice-Hall.

Kimmel, D. (1978). Adult development and aging: A gay perspective. *Journal of Social Issues, 34,* 113–130.

Kinsey, A. C., Pomeroy, W. B., & Martin, C. E. (1948). *Sexual behavior in the human male.* Philadelphia: W. B. Saunders.

Kinsey, A. C., Pomeroy, W. B., Martin, C. E., & Gebhard, P. H. (1953). *Sexual behavior in the human female.* Philadelphia: W. B. Saunders.

Kirkpatrick, M., & Morgan, C. (1980). Psychodynamic psychotherapy of female homosexuality. In J. Marmor (Ed.), *Homosexual behavior: A modern reappraisal* (pp. 357–375). New York: Basic Books.

Klein, F., Sepekoff, B., & Wolf, T. J. (1985). Sexual orientation: A multivariable dynamic process. *Journal of Homosexuality, 11,* 35–49.

Koodin, H., Morin, S., Riddle, D., Rogers, M., Sang, B., & Strassburger, F. (1979). *Removing the stigma. Final report. Task force on the status of lesbian and gay male psychologists.* Washington, DC: American Psychological Association.

Krieger, S. (1982). Lesbian identity and community: Recent social science literature. *Signs, 8,* 91–108.

Kwawer, J. S. (1980). Transference and countertransference in homosexuality—changing psychoanalytic views. *American Journal of Psychotherapy, 34,* 72–80.

Larson, P. C. (1981). Sexual identity and self-concept. *Journal of Homosexuality, 7,* 15–32.

La Torre, R. A., & Wendenburg, K. (1983). Psychological characteristics of bisexual, heterosexual, and homosexual women. *Journal of Homosexuality, 9,* 87–97.

Lee, J. A. (1977). Going public: A study in the sociology of homosexual liberation. *Journal of Homosexuality, 3,* 47–78.

Legier, D. (1986). Patterns of diversity among homosexual and heterosexual women. *Dissertation Abstracts International, 46,* 4018B.

Lewes, K. (1988). *Power to hurt: The psychoanalytic theory of male homosexuality.* New York: Simon & Schuster.

Liazos, A. (1980). The poverty of the sociology of deviance: Nuts, sluts, and "preverts." In S. H. Traub & C. B. Little (Eds.), *Theories of deviance* (pp. 330–352). Itasca, IL: F. E. Peacock.

Lipsitz, J. (1977). *Growing up forgotten.* Lexington, MA: Lexington Books.

Loney, J. (1972). Background factors, sexual experiences, and attitudes toward treatment in two "normal" homosexual samples. *Journal of Consulting and Clinical Psychology, 38,* 57–65.

Lutz, D., Roback, H., & Hart, M. (1984). Feminine gender identity and psychological adjustment of male-transsexuals and male homosexuals. *Journal of Sex Research, 20,* 350–362.

MacDonald, G. B. (1983, December). Exploring sexual identity: Gay people and their families. *Sex Education Coalition News, 5* (4), 1, 4.

Magee, B. (1966). *One in twenty.* New York: Stein & Day.

Mallen, C. A. (1983). Sex role stereotypes, gender identity and parental relationships in male homosexuals and heterosexuals. *Journal of Homosexuality, 9,* 55–74.

Malyon, A. K. (1981). The homosexual adolescent: Developmental issues and social bias. *Child Welfare, 60,* 321–330.

Manosevitz, M. (1970). Early sexual behavior in adult homosexual and heterosexual males. *Journal of Abnormal Psychology, 76,* 396–402.

Martin, A. D. (1982). Learning to hide: The socialization of the gay adolescent. *Adolescent Psychiatry, 10,* 52–65.

Maslow, A. H. (1954). *Motivation and personality.* New York: Harper.

McDonald, G. J. (1982). Individual differences in the coming out process for gay men: Implications for theoretical models. *Journal of Homosexuality, 8,* 47–60.

McDonald, G. J. (1984). Identity congruency and identity management among gay men. *Dissertation Abstracts International, 45,* 1322B.

McIntosh, M. (1968). The homosexual role. *Social Problems, 16,* 182–192.

McKirnan, D. J., & Peterson, P. L. (1986, October 2). Preliminary social issues survey results. *Windy City Times,* pp. 2, 8.

McKirnan, D. J., & Peterson, P. L. (1987a, March 12). Chicago survey documents anti-gay bias. *Windy City Times,* pp. 1, 2, 12.

McKirnan, D. J., & Peterson, P. L. (1987b, April 30). Social support and coping resources. *Windy City Times,* pp. 1, 8, 9.

McKirnan, D. J., & Peterson, P. L. (1987c, June 25). A profile of older gay males: A perspective from the social issues survey. *Windy City Times,* pp. 20, 22.

McWhirter, D. P., & Mattison, A. M. (1984). *The male couple: How relationships develop.* Englewood Cliffs, NJ: Prentice-Hall.

Mead, G. H. (1934). *Mind, self and society.* Chicago: University of Chicago Press.

Mervis, M. (1985). A comparison of lesbians and heterosexual women on the Rorschach. *Dissertation Abstracts International, 45,* 3625B.

Miller, B. (1978). Adult sexual resocialization. *Alternative Lifestyles, 1,* 207–234.

Miranda, J. (1986, August). *Evaluation of DSM-III ego-dystonic homosexuality.* Paper presented at the annual meeting of the American Psychological Association, Washington, DC.

Morin, S. F., & Garfinkle, E. M. (1978). Male homophobia. *Journal of Social Issues, 34,* 29–47.

Money, J., & Ehrhardt, A. A. (1972). *Man and woman, boy and girl.* Baltimore, MD: Johns Hopkins University Press.

Moses, A. E., & Buckner, J. A. (1980). The special problems of rural gay clients. *Human Services in the Rural Environment, 5,* 22–27.

Muchmore, W., & Hanson, W. (Eds.). (1982). *Coming out right: A handbook for the gay male.* Boston: Alyson.

Murdoch, J. (1988, October 24). Gay youths' deadly despair: High rate of suicide attempts tracked. *Washington Post,* pp. A1 & A10.

Myrick, F. L. (1974a). Homosexual types: An empirical investigation. *Journal of Sex Research, 10,* 226–237.

Myrick, F. L. (1974b). Attitudinal differences between heterosexually and homosexually oriented males and between covert and overt male homosexuals. *Journal of Abnormal Psychology, 83,* 81–86.

Naylor, G. (1982). *The women of Brewster Place.* New York: Viking.

Nemeyer, L. (1980). Coming out: Identity congruence and the attainment of adult female sexuality. *Dissertation Abstracts International, 41,* 1924B.

Nietzsche, F. (1961). *Thus spoke Zarathustra.* Baltimore, MD: Penguin.

Nottelmann, E. D., Susman, E. J., Dorn, L. D., Inoff-Germain, G., Loriaux, D. L., Cutler, G. B., Jr., & Chrousos, G. P. (1987). Developmental processes in early adolescence: Relations among chronological age, pubertal stage, height, weight, and serum levels of gonadotropins, sex steroids, and adrenal androgens. *Journal of Adolescent Health Care, 8,* 246–260.

Nungesser, L. G. (1983). *Homosexual acts, actors, and identities.* New York: Praeger.

O'Carolan, R. J. (1982). An investigation of the relationship of self-disclosure of sexual preference to self-esteem, feminism, and locus of control in lesbians. *Dissertation Abstracts International, 43,* 915B.

Ogg, E. (1978). *Changing views of homosexuality.* New York: Public Affairs Committee.

Ohlson, E., & Wilson, M. (1974). Differentiating female homosexuals from female heterosexuals by use of the MMPI. *Journal of Sex Research, 10,* 308–315.

Openshaw, D. K., Thomas, D. L., & Rollins, B. C. (1984). Parental influences of adolescent self-esteem. *Journal of Early Adolescence, 4,* 259–274.

Ovesey, L. (1965). Pseudohomosexuality and homosexuality in men: Psychodynamics as a guide to treatment. In J. Marmor (Ed.), *Sexual inversion: The multiple roots of homosexuality* (pp. 211–233). New York: Basic Books.

Ovesey, L., & Woods, S. M. (1980). Pseudohomosexuality and homosexuality in men: Psychodynamics as a guide to treatment. In J. Marmor (Ed.), *Homosexual behavior: A modern reappraisal* (pp. 325–341). New York: Basic Books.

Paul, W. (1982). Minority status for gay people: Majority reaction and social context. In W. Paul, J. D. Weinrich, J. C. Gonsiorek, & M. E. Hotvedt (Eds.), *Homosexuality: Social, psychological, and biological issues* (pp. 351–369). Beverly Hills, CA: Sage.

Pennington, M. B. (1983). Vocation discernment and the homosexual. In R. Nugent (Ed.), *A challenge to love: Gay and lesbian Catholics in the church* (pp. 235–244). New York: Crossroad.

Peterson, R. W. (1988, February 14). Seattle report: School is tough for young gays. *The Advocate*, p. 15.

Peterson, R. W. (1989a, January 17). Taking risks at Mead High. *The Advocate*, pp. 12–13.

Peterson, R. W. (1989b, April 11). In harm's way. *The Advocate*, pp. 8–10.

Picciotto, S. R. (1984). Marital satisfaction in stable gay couples. *Dissertation Abstracts International, 45*, 1028B.

Playboy Panel. (1971). Homosexuality: A symposium on the causes and consequences, social and psychological, of sexual inversion. *Playboy, 18*(4), 61f.

Plummer, K. (1975). *Sexual stigma: An interactionist account.* Boston: Routledge & Kegan Paul.

Plummer, K. (1981). *The makings of the modern homosexual.* London: Hutchison.

Ponse, B. (1980). Lesbians and their worlds. In J. Marmor (Ed.), *Homosexual behavior: A modern reappraisal* (pp. 157–175). New York: Basic Books.

Price, J. H. (1982). High school students' attitudes toward homosexuality. *Journal of School Health, 52*, 469–474.

Prytula, R. E., Wellford, C. D., & DeMonbreun, B. G. (1979). Body self-image and homosexuality. *Journal of Clinical Psychology, 35*, 567–572.

Ramsey, G. V. (1973). The sexual development of boys. *American Journal of Psychiatry, 56*, 217–234.

Raphael, S. M., & Robinson, M. K. (1980). The older lesbian: Love relationships and friendship patterns. *Alternative Lifestyles, 3*, 207–229.

Rector, P. K. (1982). The acceptance of a homosexual identity in adolescence: A phenomenological study. *Dissertation Abstracts International, 43*, 883B.

Reiche, R., & Dannecker, M. (1977). Male homosexuality in West Germany—A sociological investigation. *Journal of Sex Research, 13*, 35–53.

Reinisch, J. M., & Sanders, S. A. (1984). Prenatal gonadal steroidal influences on gender-related behavior. *Progress in Brain Research, 61*, 407–416.

Remafedi, G. (1987a). Male homosexuality: The adolescent's perspective. *Pediatrics, 79*, 326–330.

Remafedi, G. (1987b). Adolescent homosexuality: Psychosocial and medical implications. *Pediatrics, 79*, 331–337.

Richardson, D. (1981a). Theoretical perspectives on homosexuality. In J. Hart & D. Richardson (Eds.), *The theory and practice of homosexuality* (pp. 5–37). London: Routledge & Kegan Paul.

Richardson, D. (1981b). Lesbian identities. In J. Hart & D. Richardson (Eds.), *The theory and practice of homosexuality* (pp. 111–124). London: Routledge & Kegan Paul.

Riddle, D. I., & Morin, S. F. (Eds.). (1978). Psychology and the gay community. *Journal of Social Issues, 34*, 1–138.

Rigg, C. A. (1982). Homosexuality in adolescence. *Pediatric Annals, 11*, 826–829.

Robertson, R. (1981). Young gays. In J. Hart & D. Richardson (Eds.), *The theory and practice of homosexuality* (pp. 170–176). London: Routledge & Kegan Paul.

Robinson, G. (1984). Few solutions for a young dilemma. *The Advocate*, pp. 14–16.

Robinson, L. H. (1980). Adolescent homosexual patterns: Psychodynamics and therapy. *Adolescent Psychiatry, 8*, 422–433.

Rodriguez, R. A. (1988, August). *Significant events in gay identity development: Gay men in Utah.* Paper presented at the annual meeting of the American Psychological Association, Atlanta, GA.

Roesler, T., & Deisher, R. (1972). Youthful male homosexuality. *Journal of the American Medical Association, 219*, 1018–1023.

Rofes, E. E. (1984, November 27). Youth: New identities, new issue. *The Advocate*, pp. 30–31.

Romm, M. E. (1965). Sexuality and homosexuality in women. In J. Marmor (Ed.), *Sexual inversion: The multiple roots of homosexuality* (pp. 282–301). New York: Basic Books.

Rosenberg, M. (1965). *Society and the adolescent self-image.* Princeton, NJ: Princeton University Press.

Rosenberg, M. (1979). *Conceiving the self.* New York: Basic Books.

Ross, M. W. (1980). Retrospective distortion in homosexual research. *Archives of Sexual Behavior, 9*, 523–531.

Ross-Reynolds, G. (1982). Issues in counseling the "homosexual" adolescent. In J. Grimes (Ed.), *Psychological approaches to problems of children and adolescents* (pp. 55–88). Des Moines: Iowa State Department of Education.

Russo, V. (1987). *The celluloid closet.* New York: Harper & Row.

Rutter, M. (1987). Psychosocial resilience and protective mechanisms. *American Journal of Orthopsychiatry, 57*, 316–331.

Sagarin, E., & Kelly, R. J. (1980). Sexual deviance and labelling perspectives. In W. R. Gove (Ed.), *The labelling of deviance: Evaluating a perspective* (pp. 347–379). New York: Sage.

Saghir, M. T., & Robins, E. (1969). Homosexuality: I. Sexual behavior of the female homosexual. *Archives of General Psychiatry, 20*, 192–201.

Saghir, M. T., & Robins, E. (1973). *Male and female homosexuality.* Baltimore, MD: Williams & Wilkins.

Saghir, M. T., & Robins, E. (1980). Clinical aspects of female homosexuality. In J. Marmor (Ed.), *Homosexual behavior: A modern reappraisal* (pp. 280–295). New York: Basic Books.

Saghir, M. T., & Robins, E., & Walbran, B. (1969). Homosexuality: II. Sexual behavior of the male homosexual. *Archives of General Psychiatry, 21*, 219–229.

Sanders, D. S. (1980). A psychotherapeutic approach to homosexual men. In J. Marmor (Ed.), *Homosexual behavior: A modern reappraisal* (pp. 342–356). New York: Basic Books.

Sanders, G. (1980). Homosexualities in the Netherlands. *Alternative Lifestyles, 3*, 278–311.

Sandfort, T. G. M. (1983). Pedophile relationships in the Netherlands: Alternative lifestyle for children? *Alternative Lifestyles, 5*, 164–183.

Sang, B. E. (1978). Lesbian research: A critical evaluation. In G. Vida (Ed.), *Our right to love: A lesbian resource book* (pp. 80–87). Englewood Cliffs, NJ: Prentice-Hall.

Savin-Williams, R. C. (1987a). *Adolescence: An ethological perspective.* New York: Springer-Verlag.

Savin-Williams, R. C. (1987b). An ethological perspective on homosexuality during adolescence. *Journal of Adolescent Research, 2*, 283–302.

Savin-Williams, R. C. (1989a). Parental influences on the self-esteem of gay and lesbian youths: A reflected appraisals model. *Journal of Homosexuality, 17*, 93–109.

Savin-Williams, R. C. (1989b). Coming out to parents and self-esteem among gay and lesbian youths. *Journal of Homosexuality, 18*, 1–35.

Savin-Williams, R. C. (1989c). *The attitudes of "privileged" adolescents toward homosexuality.* Manuscript in preparation.

Savin-Williams, R. C., & Berndt, T. J. (1990). Friendships and peer relations. In S. S. Feldman & G. R. Elliott (Eds.), *At the threshold: The developing adolescent.* Cambridge, MA: Harvard University Press.

Savin-Williams, R. C., & Demo, D. H. (1983a). Conceiving or misconceiving the self: Issues in adolescent self-esteem. *Journal of Early Adolescence, 3*, 121–140.

Savin-Williams, R. C., & Demo, D. H. (1983b). Situational and transituational determinants of adolescent self-feelings. *Journal of Personality and Social Psychology, 44*, 832–841.

Savin-Williams, R. C., & Demo, D. H. (1984). Developmental change and stability in adolescent self-concept. *Developmental Psychology, 20*, 1100–1110.

Savin-Williams, R. C., & Jaquish, G. A. (1981). The assessment of adolescent self-esteem. A comparison of methods. *Journal of Personality, 49*, 324–336.

Savin-Williams, R. C., & Weisfeld, G. E. (1989). An ethological perspective on adolescence. In G. R. Adams, R. Montemayer, & T. P. Gullotta (Eds.), *Biology of adolescent behavior and development* (pp. 249–274). Newbury Park, CA: Sage.

Schafer, S. (1976). Sexual and social problems of lesbians. *Journal of Sex Research, 12*, 50–69.

Schafer, S. (1977). Sociosexual behavior in male and female homosexuals: A study in sex differences. *Archives of Sexual Behavior, 6*, 355–364.

Schofield, M. (1965). *Sociological aspects of homosexuality.* Boston: Little, Brown.

Schwanberg, S. L. (1985). Changes in labeling homosexuality in health sciences literature: A preliminary investigation. *Journal of Homosexuality, 12*, 51–73.

Shively, M. G., & DeCecco, J. P. (1977). Components of sexual identity. *Journal of Homosexuality, 3*, 41–48.

Shively, M. G., Jones, C., & DeCecco, J. P. (1983/1984). Research on sexual orientation: Definitions and models. *Journal of Homosexuality, 9*, 127–136.

Siegelman, M. (1972a). Adjustment of homosexual and heterosexual women. *British Journal of Psychiatry, 120*, 477–481.

Siegelman, M. (1972b). Adjustment of male homosexuals and heterosexuals. *Archives of Sexual Behavior, 2*, 9–25.

Siegelman, M. (1978). Psychological adjustment of homosexual and heterosexual men: A cross-national replication. *Archives of Sexual Behavior, 7*, 1–11.

Siegelman, M. (1979). Adjustment of homosexual and heterosexual women: A cross-national replication. *Archives of Sexual Behavior, 8,* 121–125.

Silverstein, C. (1977). *Family matters: A parents' guide to homosexuality.* New York: McGraw-Hill.

Silverstein, C. (1981). *Man to man: Gay couples in America.* New York: Quill.

Simmons, R. G., & Blyth, D. A. (1987). *Moving into adolescence: The impact of pubertal change and school context.* Hawthorne, NY: Aldine deGruyter.

Simon, W., & Gagnon, J. H. (1967). Homosexuality: The formulation of a sociological perspective. *Journal of Health and Social Behavior, 8,* 177–185.

Skrapec, C., & MacKenzie, K. R. (1981). Psychological self-perception in male transsexuals, homosexuals, and heterosexuals. *Archives of Sexual Behavior, 10,* 357–369.

Smith, T. A. (1983). Sexual identity and reproductive motivations. *Dissertation Abstracts International, 44,* 1979B.

Sobel, H. J. (1976). Adolescent attitudes toward homosexuality in relation to self-concept and body satisfaction. *Adolescence, 11,* 443–453.

Socarides, C. W. (1968). *The overt homosexual.* London: Grune & Stratton.

Solnit, A. J. (1969). Bisexuality gone away: The child is father to the man. *Pediatrics, 43,* 913–914.

Sophie, J. (1985/1986). A critical examination of stage theories of lesbian identity development. *Journal of Homosexuality, 12,* 39–51.

Sorensen, R. (1973). *Adolescent sexuality in contemporary society.* New York: World Book.

Spada, J. (1979). *The Spada Report: The newest survey of gay male sexuality.* New York: New American Library.

Spence, J. T., & Helmreich, R. L. (1978). *Masculinity and femininity: Their psychological dimensions, correlates, and antecedents.* Austin, TX: University of Texas Press.

Stanley, J. P., & Wolfe, S. J. (Eds.). (1980). *The coming out stories.* New York: Persephone.

Stekel, W. (1922). *The homosexual neurosis.* Brooklyn, NY: Physicians and Surgeons.

Storms, M. D. (1980). Theories of sexual orientation. *Journal of Personality and Social Psychology, 38,* 783–792.

Storms, M. D. (1981). A theory of erotic orientation development. *Psychological Review, 88,* 340–353.

Strassberg, D. S., Roback, H., Cunningham, J., McKee, E., & Larson, P. (1979). Psychopathology in self-identified female-to-male transsexuals, homosexuals, and heterosexuals. *Archives of Sexual Behavior, 8,* 491–496.

Straver, C. J. (1976). Research on homosexuality in the Netherlands. *The Netherlands' Journal of Sociology, 12,* 121–137.

Sullivan, H. S. (1953). *The interpersonal theory of psychiatry.* New York: Norton.

Suppe, F. (1984). In defense of a multidimensional approach to sexual identity. *Journal of Homosexuality, 10,* 7–14.

Tannahill, R. (1980). *Sex in history.* New York: Stein & Day.

Thompson, N. (1973). Parent child relationships and sexual identity in male and female homosexuals and heterosexuals. *Journal of Counseling and Clinical Psychology, 41,* 120–127.

Thompson, N. L., McCandless, B. R., & Strickland, B. R. (1971). Personal adjustment of male and female homosexuals and heterosexuals. *Journal of Abnormal Psychology, 78,* 237–240.

Tripp, C. A. (1975). *The homosexual matrix.* New York: McGraw-Hill.

Troiden, R. R. (1979). Becoming homosexual: A model of gay identity acquisition. *Psychiatry, 42,* 362–373.

Troiden, R. R. (1989). The formation of homosexual identities. *Journal of Homosexuality, 17,* 43–73.

Uhrig, L. J. (1984). *The two of us: Affirming, celebrating and symbolizing gay and lesbian relationships.* Boston: Alyson.

VanWyk, P. H., & Geist, C. S. (1984). Psychosocial development of heterosexual, bisexual, and homosexual behavior. *Archives of Sexual Behavior, 13,* 505–544.

Vergara, T. L. (1983/1984). Meeting the needs of sexual minority youth: One program's response. *Journal of Social Work & Human Sexuality, 2,* 19–38.

Vining, D. (1988, January 5). Rediscovering our history: Don't forget the gay times. *The Advocate,* p. 9.

Warren, C. (1974). *Identity and community in the gay world.* New York: John Wiley.

Warren, C. (1977). Fieldwork in the gay world: Issues in phenomenological research. *Journal of Social Issues, 33,* 93–107.

Wayson, P. D. (1985). Personality variables in males as they relate to differences in sexual orientation. *Journal of Homosexuality, 11,* 63–73.

Weinberg, G. (1972). *Society and the healthy homosexual.* New York: St. Martin.

Weinberg, M. S., & Bell, A. P. (Eds.). (1972). *Homosexuality: An annotated bibliography.* New York: Harper & Row.

Weinberg, M. S., & Williams, C. J. (1974). *Male homosexuals: Their problems and adaptations.* New York: Penguin.

Weinberg, T. S. (1978). On "doing" and "being" gay: Sexual behavior and homosexual male self-identity. *Journal of Homosexuality, 4,* 143–156.

Weinberg, T. S. (1983). *Gay men, gay selves.* New York: Irvington.

Weis, C. B., Jr., & Dain, R. N. (1979). Ego development and sex attitude in heterosexual and homosexual men and women. *Archives of Sexual Behavior, 8,* 341–356.

West, D. J. (1967). *Homosexuality.* Chicago: Aldine.

Westmoreland, C. (1975). A study of long-term relationships among male homosexuals. *Dissertation Abstracts International, 36,* 3132B.

Whitam, F. L. (1977). The homosexual role: A reconsideration. *Journal of Sex Research, 13,* 1–11.

Whitam, F. L. (1983). Culturally invariable properties of male homosexuality: Tentative conclusions from cross-cultural research. *Archives of Sexual Behavior, 12,* 207–226.

Whitam, F. L., & Mathy, R. M. (1987). *Male homosexuality in four societies: Brazil, Guatemala, the Philippines, and the United States.* New York: Praeger.

White, E. (1982). *A boy's own story.* New York: E. P. Dutton.

Wiesen, S. C. (1987, February 12). Mythcontheptions about being gay. *Montclair Kimberley Academy News* (Montclair, NJ), Vol. XIII, Issue 4, p. 2.

Wilkins, J. L. (1981). A comparative study of male homosexual personality factors: Brief cruising encounters vs. ongoing relationships. *Dissertation Abstracts International, 42,* 2555B.

Wilson, M. (1987, April 16). Frontlines: Coming out to new perspectives. *Windy City Times,* p. 8.

Wilson, M., & Greene, R. (1971). Personality characteristics of female homosexuals. *Psychological Reports, 28,* 407–412.

Wong, M. J. (1980). Long-term homosexual and heterosexual couple relationship effects on self-concept and relationship adjustment. *Dissertation Abstracts International, 41,* 1169B.

Woodman, N. J., & Lenna, H. R. (1980). *Counseling with gay men and women.* San Francisco: Jossey-Bass.

Youman, R. (1985, November 10). Making contact. *New York Times Magazine,* p. 74.

Zuger, B. (1978). Effeminate behavior present in boys from childhood: Ten additional years of follow-up. *Comprehensive Psychiatry, 19,* 363–369.

Index